Secrets of Growing Young

SECRETS OF GROWING YOUNG

by Anthony Barker

DRAKE PUBLISHERS INC NEW YORK

ISBN 0-87749-279-4
LCCCN 72-2448

Published in 1973 by
Drake Publishers Inc
381 Park Avenue South
New York, N.Y. 10016

Printed in the United States of America

Contents

There Has Never Been A Better Time For Growing Young

This book is written for men and women of all ages who are more interested in enjoying their years than in counting them.

It tells how to toss aside the old life-denying myths that make second-class citizens of the over-thirty woman, the over-forty man, and the over-fifty couple and how to achieve a full emotional, sexual, social, and creative life—the one sure way to keep "youthfully fresh in body, mind, or feeling," which is Webster's definition of "young."

It tells how to establish contact with the life-renewing forces within and how to make them work for you. And it tells how to conquer those enemies of a long, joyous, and rewarding life: psychological fatigue, boredom, destructive routine, and fear of living one's life to the fullest.

Thanks to medical science and technology, the prospect of a longer life increasingly opens out before us. Yet mentally and physically we remain prisoners of the negative habits and life styles that bring on premature age.

It is time we realized that whether we are thirty-five, forty-five, fifty-five or sixty-five, change, growth, a more youthful appearance, a more fulfilling and exciting existence are not only possible today but are within reach of practically all of us, and without recourse to pills or magic potions.

Whatever our age, that frequently repeated sigh, "It's too late now," no longer offers a valid excuse for avoiding the challenge of life. For each of us possesses more than enough renewal energy to transform our lives, starting today, and as never before, society invites us to use it in grow-young ways.

Learning to tap that source of youthful energy can provide us with some of the most enjoyable experiences of our lives. And whether we are trimming off pounds, involving ourselves with new friends and projects, or venturing a different life style, the most effective actions are those we enter into joyously.

At one time, facing the challenge of change after thirty was truly a formidable task, Fortunately, we live in a time when liberating change swirls about every aspect of our lives, whether we are teen-agers or grandparents, so that we can confidently say, "There has never been a better time for growing young."

Everywhere the old stereotypes that forced us into the molds of premature age are crumbling. We no longer believe that we have to be married by thirty, can't switch careers once we have reached forty, that bright colors and gay fashions are out after fifty, and that sexual fulfillment is rare after sixty. We know better. In food, clothing, places to live, personal relations, jobs, interests, the choices are as wide as our desires. Each of us can grow young in our own way.

With the air cleared of old-fashioned and misleading myths, we can start to get a new and healthier perspective on our lives and learn to accept our imperfections and idiosyncrasies—and potentialities—as integral parts of that unique, irreplaceable, and wondrous self from which all energy flows.

From acceptance we move on to change, taking charge of our lives and channeling our energy toward youthful goals. And not with grim exercises and harsh disciplines but with pleasurable grow-young activities, we set ourselves on the new course that is uniquely our own.

The time to begin is now, today. "Just over thirty" is a great age to start your grow-young program. So is "just over fifty." Because it is never too late for you.

The activities and programs in this book are within reach of practically everyone. They build confidence by leading from one success to another. And they fit into the scheme of the everyday, workaday world we all inhabit.

They are also enjoyable, exhilarating, rewarding. The element of pleasure, stressed throughout the book, is not just an afterthought included to make the programs more attractive. Joyous activity is basic to the entire concept of growing young. The more you use this book to open your mind and senses to pleasurable and rewarding experiences, the faster your grow-young efforts will produce results.

There are more activities and projects included than you can absorb at once. But in developing a youthful spirit and personality, in achieving a more attractive and striking appearance, "variety is the spice of life." With variety you can suit your mood of the moment or overcome the limitations of a particular situation and still carry on your grow-young program uninterrupted. And, what is most important of all, variety recognizes the uniqueness of you.

There are many paths to growing young in this book. Test. Experiment. Combine. And joyously enter into the activities and programs that release your marvelous energy for life.

How to begin?

With the "easy starters" on the following page.

Easy Starters

Here's an easy, enjoyable way to get started on your grow-young program.

Most of us must overcome a built-in resistance to change before we can begin any new project. If we fear to fail, thinking the difficulties greater than our powers, the resistance may grow insurmountable. So we do nothing.

Or we attempt to plunge right into major renovation, which is like expecting to win a mile race or qualify for entry in the tennis finals without first getting into shape. Of course we lose and become discouraged. Failed again!

But it is not our powers that are lacking. We have simply taken the wrong approach to getting started.

Begin the Easy Way

The "easy starters" in this chapter overcome resistance to change by limbering up our attitudes and breaking the aging habits into which we all fall at one time or another. And while you practice these "easy starters," they condition you for the more vigorous action ahead.

Don't underestimate their importance just because they seem so easy. They are important agents for change—and agents for change will continue to play vital roles throughout your grow-young program.

Don't be afraid to enjoy them. One of the many acquaintances to whom I have recommended the "easy starters" objected, "But this is so much fun"—as though action to change our lives had to be laborious, distasteful, and grim to be effective!

Fifteen-Minute Easy Starters

Here are over seventy-five "easy starters" designed to ease you into change. Not one of them demands more than fifteen minutes of your time. You don't need to attempt all of them at once. But aim at practicing at least one each day for two weeks.

Comb your hair in a different way. Experiment with a new style and give it a chance before returning to the old—if you do.

Try a food new to you—persimmon, mango, okra, leeks, eggplant, oysters.

Say "no." For once turn down the invitation you always accepted out of habit or politeness.

Talk to a stranger—at work, at a concert, in the checkout lane at the supermarket.

Paint your toenails bright red—or some other color you have never tried.

Read a modern poem, the same one three times silently and three times aloud.

Get up fifteen minutes earlier. Eat breakfast from a tray by your favorite window.

Tell off a boor—or whoever has been nagging you.

Write a quickie note to Cousin Herman and send him the old snapshot made when he was a baby.

Feed the birds.

Fulfill a childhood wish—sit through a movie three times, build a sand castle, watch the ants work.

Dress for dinner as though you were expecting your favorite "glamor person."

Spend fifteen minutes browsing in a section of the library you have always ignored.

For a change, don't put anything on your potato except salt: Enjoy the real taste of a potato.

Make a list of all the things you like most in your life.

Share your flower garden: take bouquets to a lonely old person, to your local hospital.

Make a list of changes you would make in your community—or the world—if you had the talent, time, money, courage, power.

Write an indignant letter to your local government.

Play tick tack toe with someone fifteen years older than you are—or with a child.

Sit in a place where you can watch people passing by. Observe how they walk, wear their clothes, jostle or ignore each other.

Make up a guest list for your ideal party, leaving out some of the regulars and adding others you barely know.

Listen to the sound of your own voice during a telephone conversation. Make notes on enunciation, tone, vitality, enthusiasm—the vocal image you project to others.

Plant petunias or geraniums in a window box.

Go to the circus—or a rock concert.

Make a list of the physical ailments or diseases you sometimes wonder you may have.

Write to a large diagnostic medical clinic or university

hospital about their preventive medical examinations and testing programs.

Check your telephone book for Weight Watchers or other reducing groups. Make an appointment to observe a meeting.

See if you can rub your head with one hand while patting your stomach with another.

Stop fingering your face or hair—or consciously refrain from your most pronounced nervous habit. (See: You have proved you could stop for fifteen minutes; tomorrow stop for twenty minutes; the next day for thirty; and so on.)

Take your trousers or slacks to the tailor and tell him to correct the fit.

Try on several wigs or toupees.

Go to an old Maurice Chevalier movie.

Get up early one morning. Seek solitude and peace in a church or deserted place before anyone else arrives.

Build a terrarium—or buy one ready-made.

Do nothing but listen to the sounds about you—the wind, birds, the traffic, the neighbor's vacuum cleaner. Think only of the sound.

Wear a flower in your buttonhole—or at your wrist.

Put a pinch of curry in your sandwich spread.

Read every editorial in today's newspaper and examine the reasons for your negative or positive reactions.

Tell your wife/husband that she/he is wonderful.

Move a piece of furniture to a different location.

Let someone know you need him. Ask a friend, colleague, neighbor for advice.

Offer to teach a teen-ager your favorite dance steps.

Substitute honey for sugar in your tea.

Start a button collection, beginning with those you have on hand.

Offer to walk your neighbor's dog.

Tell someone that he/she looks particularly good today.

Buy a bright blue browalia plant to bloom in your window. Or grow one from seed and give the extras away.

Follow the movement of a cloud for fifteen minutes—try to think only of the cloud.

Tell your son or daughter that he/she is improving—as a driver, speaker, a more considerate person.

Visit an antique shop. You will learn the values of those things you take for granted at home.

Serve dinner by candlelight. If your husband grouses, put one candle beside his plate so he won't doubt what he is getting. (It's a good idea to serve a familiar dish the first time).

Give your wife or girl friend a bottle of perfume.

Plan a trip to the three places in the world you consider most beautiful.

Return that book (or hammer or shovel) to its owner.

Resolve to see every film made by your favorite director.

Unplug the television set—or pretend it is out of order.

Visit a pet shop with a neighbor's child.

Gently remind a young mother not to shout at her children.

See how many new things you can learn in fifteen minutes from the dictionary or encyclopedia. Make notes.

Rehang that picture so it is only ten inches above the top of the sofa.

Sit in the early-morning sun and concentrate on the sensation caused by the sun's rays penetrating your skin.

Ask a neighbor's teen-ager if you can borrow his records one afternoon.

Make a face at yourself in the bathroom mirror—now another, as many as you can devise. Now see how good a big smile feels.

Roll your head around, from right to left and from left to right. Now let it drop as far as it will go. Notice how your muscles relax. Resolve to do this every day.

Try to imitate your favorite old-time movie star—in walk, speech, bearing.

Put grated cheese or garlic croutons on your most humdrum vegetable.

Take a couple of your brightest colored towels and a few safety pins. Drape, tie, and pin them on yourself in the most ridiculous ways you can imagine—as diapers, a halter top, a toga, skirt with slits to the waist, a face veil below the eyes, a train. Put on a show for your husband, wife—or someone you enjoy.

Lower your voice by two octaves. Keep it low for every word you speak for fifteen minutes.

Count the stars. If you live in the city, search for the big dipper; if in the country, find the milky way.

Read a magazine with a political slant different from your own.

Eat in a different location, whether at home or in a restaurant.

Challenge a teen-ager to play checkers—and let the teen win at least one game.

Read the twenty-third psalm.

> Make a list of the three things that weigh most heavily on your conscience. Write letters to the people involved. Now tear them up.

Go back and put a check by all the "easy starters" that made you feel good during or after performing them. Plan to make them a regular part of your life.

Now what has this mixed bag of "easy starters" to do with achieving a youthful mind and body?

Everything.

These actions set flowing through your system the natural renewal energy that has been blocked by the negative habits of premature aging.

They supply the necessary ingredient of confidence in your ability to change.

Once you have performed at least one of these "easy starters" each day for two weeks, no one can tell you that change is not possible. You know better because you have succeeded in making change work.

You now realize that what you have taken to be the fixed and irreversible course of your days is not fixed at all—that tomorrow can be different.

What's more, you have learned that action for change can be enjoyable, bringing its own immediate rewards as well as long-term gains.

This is an important lesson to remember throughout your grow-young program. Whether you are trimming off unwanted pounds, conquering shyness, or venturing a new life style, the most effective actions will be those you enter into joyously.

Change is the force that breaks the destructive habits of premature age. You are already well on your way to using this force to achieve your goals.

You are now ready to bring the magic of change into your life in bigger and more enduring ways.

Overcoming Roadblocks

Everyone's path is strewn with roadblocks to growing young.

Not just yours.

Not just mine.

Everyone's.

Often we can't even describe these obstacles. We just sense their looming presence and decide they are more than we can cope with. *That* road is impassable. So we do nothing, defeated before we start.

It's That Easy

Actually, the roadblocks often roll aside quite easily. Upon close examination, some of them turn out to be nothing but figments of our imagination. Even seemingly formidable ones yield to intelligent maneuvering on our part.

The first step is to locate the particular obstruction blocking your way.

The second is to roll up your sleeves and get it out of the road without further delay.

Then get on with your grow-young program.

Yes, it's that easy.

THE MOST COMMON ROADBLOCKS TO GROWING YOUNG AND WHAT TO DO ABOUT THEM.

The Blues

Presidents and prime ministers, assembly line workers and young mothers, secretaries and executives—we all get the blues at one time or another. When they hit us after thirty-five, however, we read them as signs of creeping age, indicators that our zest for life is draining away. So there's a beautiful sunset or a great new movie, who cares? Good posture, good eating habits, keeping up with the new fashions—nothing seems worth the bother. It's all blah.

WHAT TO DO ABOUT THE BLUES

> Break the mood with strenuous activity. Force yourself into the shower. Put on your most colorful togs. Go for a brisk walk. (Don't saunter this time.) Treat yourself to dinner out, a movie, a concert, a hockey game. When you get home, have a cup of tea or a glass of sherry and spend an hour planning—to take a trip, start a garden, redecorate your home, enroll in a class on some esoteric subject. Then sink into bed, fully exhausted, the mood broken.

Looking Backward

Spending our days regretting the road not taken is a sure invitation to premature age. We think of the career we might have had, the person we might have married, the great artist we might have been . . . if only! Conceding that all the big choices have been made in the past, we need take no responsibility for making decisions today. Resignedly, we sit back and watch life flow past, untouched by its magic and its beauty.

WHAT TO DO ABOUT LOOKING BACKWARD

Stop regretting and start living. You can't do anything about yesterday. You can change tomorrow, and the next day, and the next year. First concentrate on the things you can change easily: Work on your style of dressing, arrange to meet different people, develop new interests. If overweight, start to trim off a few pounds. Then outline a plan for major change, which may involve a change of jobs or residence or going back to school. Read the section on "Easy Starters" and "The Magic of Change." Live your days, don't waste them looking back. And remember that not making a decision is in itself a decision—a decision to stay in the same old rut you're in now.

Anxiety

We worry about the loss of our youth, of our sexual appeal and prowess, of our ability to compete socially and in business, of our competence in handling the everyday affairs of life. Will I be desired, liked, accepted? Will I have enough money? Can I do the job? Am I growing old? Do I have some incurable disease? Questions like these haunt our waking hours, undermining our self-confidence and esteem and destroying our pleasure in living.

WHAT TO DO ABOUT ANXIETY

Conquer anxiety with action. There's no point in advising, "Don't be anxious about your appearance," if that's what is bothering you. But once you start doing something about your hair, posture, clothes, and so on, anxiety crumbles beneath the impact of action. Perhaps the most troublesome aspect of anxiety is the way it floats around our consciousness unmoored to any particular cause. The best antidote for free-floating anxiety is to crowd your day with meaningful and enjoyable activity. Walking, visiting old friends, sewing, macrame, woodcarving, gardening, almost any activity that demands both physical and mental involvement can serve as a good mood breaker for dispelling anxiety. (Some anxiety is normal. To be unconcerned about our fate, individually and collectively, is to be less than human. Our goal should be to prevent anxiety from reaching unmanageable proportions.)

Stress

Like anxiety, stress is a part of everyone's life. But much of it is unnecessary, self-imposed. We compete when we don't have to, we set arbitrary deadlines and impossible performance expectations. We strive always to be the best—the best housekeeper, the hardest driving executive, the superlover. Huffing and puffing we congratulate ourself, "There, I've done it!" But the pressure of ruthless schedules and exacting standards removes all pleasure in the doing. Inevitably, stress takes its emotional and bodily toll.

WHAT TO DO ABOUT STRESS

When you feel stress building up, take a break from whatever you are doing and involve yourself in some activity that gives you some rewards: hobbies, talking to a friend, working on some long-range plan. Seek out noncompetitive situations, where there are no winners or losers but just people having a good time together. If the social treadmill moves too fast, jump off. Break the stress pattern imposed by social obligations. Go off on your own. Invent an excuse: You have to go out of town—and if you can, get out of town. Spend a day at a quiet country inn or visit a museum. Get back together with yourself. (See "A Time for Quiet.") With your new perspective, the occasion for stress will fall into place as just one aspect of your life and not deserving of the importance you accorded it with worry and emotion.

Fatigue

Always tired! Not an ounce of energy left to do another thing. No wonder we feel old and dejected.

WHAT TO DO ABOUT FATIGUE

Tired, yes—but tired of what?
Of your job? Housework? The same old routine?
Unless your exhaustion is triggered by a physical cause, the cure lies not in doing less but in doing more: more of the things that give you pleasure, excitement, rewards. Housewives, for example, who complain of being bone-tired are not overstating their case. They are exhausted from doing the same thing day in and day out. Collapsing on the bed affords no relief. But break the routine with an evening out, a part-time job, an occasion to mix with new people and get onto a new energy wavelength, and watch that tired feeling vanish! Sometimes you may be too tired to take the necessary action because fatigue has been allowed to accumulate and sap your will power. Then see your doctor. He may change your diet or prescribe some energy support that will give you the initial drive to make the break from fatigue-producing routine. In any event and at all cost: Give yourself something pleasurable to look forward to. Plan it now and make a commitment to it.

"Act Your Age"

"What will people say, dating at your age?" "You must think you're a teenager, wearing that dress" (or jacket, hair style, wig, etc) . "Don't you think you should slow down a bit?" "It's too late for you to . . ."

WHAT TO DO ABOUT "ACT YOUR AGE"

Recognize the "act your age" counsel for what it is: an attempt by others to shape your life in the image of their prejudices. More than likely it's done out of fear that they will be left behind, or jealousy. Then realize that whenever you do something that rewards you with a "great to be alive" feeling, whether it's sports, collecting stamps, striding along with a perfectly outrageous walking stick, taking a job after twenty years of housework, or making love—you are acting your age. Just tell your critics that you are not living in the past and that life is meant to be lived.

Playing it Safe

Day in and day out, we rise and retire at the same hours, follow the same route to and from work, see the same people, read the same newspapers and magazines. It's all very reassuring—and deadly, hardening the mental and emotional arteries and depriving ourselves of the air and space we need to grow young.

WHAT TO DO ABOUT PLAYING IT SAFE

Take a chance. Keep in mind that after thirty the real danger lies in "settling in" and not in "branching out." Experiment with a new style of dressing. Volunteer for a community action project. Dine in a restaurant serving exotic foreign dishes. Apply for a new job. Talk to a stranger. Step outside the "playing it safe" box into the wide world and enrich your life with new and different experiences.

Segregation by Age

All our friends are our own age. Understandably, this can be comforting, since we are not jarred by the different philosophies and attitudes of the very young or the very old. In conversation, they and we know what to expect. It's dull, dull, dull.

WHAT TO DO ABOUT SEGREGATION BY AGE

Break out of the generation trap. Make an effort to get involved with people of all ages. Community action, amateur theater, politics, adult education, chess, sports, arts and crafts are just a few occasions where you will find people ranging from the twenties to the eighties, happily mingling together. Invite teenagers and older people to your home—at the same time. It will be an occasion all of you will remember instead of another ho-hum evening with the same old crowd.

Finances

"But I can't afford new clothes." "It costs a lot of money to keep up socially with people who do exciting things." "I need to save all the money I can to see me through my old age."

WHAT TO DO ABOUT FINANCES

Growing young in attitudes is free—free as the lift we get when we hear a bird singing, free as the heart when we join a small child in a dance or song, free as the spirit of the kite we fly, especially if we have a twelve-year-old as our teacher. A luxurious bath with scented soap is seldom beyond the means of any of us, nor is a new hair styling. If you have only lack of money as an excuse for dragging your feet, admit that it is more likely lack of imagination. Repairing the damage to health and spirit by failing to start a grow-young program will cost far more than the small sum required for the suggestions given in this book. Most of them require only the expenditure of faith in yourself and the knowledge that life is far too precious to be wasted in a not-living existence.

Feeling Good About Yourself

Each of us is unique, important, irreplaceable.

There are no substitutes for you, no photocopies.

Acknowledge this uniqueness in all its rich and varied colors and you have taken the essential step toward feeling good about yourself.

To have a good opinion of yourself means accepting the basic "you." That doesn't rule out change because change is a basic condition of your existence.

But it does mean allowing yourself to be different from others—and even relishing the difference.

It means focusing your energy on realizing your own potential instead of trying to conform to someone else's idea of who and what you should be.

It means putting perfection in its place. The most likable people are those who have faults—and let them show. We enjoy them because they are not continuously sending out critical vibrations. They let us be, so we relax and enjoy them, and in their presence we feel good about ourselves. So it is that in accepting ourselves we make it easier for others to accept themselves.

It is when we turn against ourselves, denying our desires, our limitations, our idiosyncrasies, our physical characteristics—our uniqueness, in short—that we set in motion the process of self-destruction. For whatever may be wrong with our present existence, it is still the vital center from which springs the energy for all of our grow-young actions.

But why do we so often reject our individuality and as a result suffer such a poor opinion of ourselves?

And, most important of all, what can we do to get a new and positive perspective?

The Enemy Within

No one can run us down as skillfully and relentlessly as we can.

Acutely aware of our shortcomings, plagued by feelings of guilt and inferiority, we fancy ourselves the world's greatest authority on what is wrong with us.

In reality, the negative image we have of ourselves is the product of innumerable distortions and misconceptions that have been accumulating since childhood.

Thus we try to conform to the expectations of others rather than develop our uniqueness.

We set impossibly high standards for ourselves, as though determined to prove that we are failures.

Instead of acting to enhance our self-esteem, we seek to buy the good opinion of others by inviting them to walk over us.

Or we continue to punish ourselves for some imagined sin we think we may have committed.

The "I am Not Worthy" Syndrome

Why are we so bent on self-destruction?

One cause is the brainwashing most of us undergo in childhood. In the mistaken belief that they are spurring us on to greater efforts, parents and teachers frequently focused attention on our shortcomings to the point where they loomed as major defects. So the failure to pass a test or to appreciate a certain food haunts us through adulthood.

Another is failure to live up to our standards. The failure may have been sexual, financial, moral, or whatever. For example, guilt may have overwhelmed us because we failed to experience what we considered adequate grief at the loss of a friend or because we broke one of the ten commandments, forgetting that religious principles also include forgiveness.

This leads to one of the major causes for running ourselves down, which may be called "Great Expectations." We live in an age of superstars—whether they be lovers, actors, writers, sports figures, tycoons, or just "beautiful people," it is against their blown-up cinematic images that we measure ourselves—and inevitably find that we are wanting. Understandably, a crippling feeling of inadequacy sets in when we compare with those projections on the giant screens of the media our own figure, IQ, earning power, orgasmic capacity, conversational brilliance, and ability to appear sparkling, desirable, cool, and collected after eight hours on the job, at home or in the office.

Then there are the "inferiority traps" set by society. If you don't have a college education, if you do have a strange accent, if you work with your hands, if you don't swing while your neighbors do—the list of situations that may induce a low opinion of ourselves, if we allow them to, is endless.

Perhaps the most prevalent of all reasons for not feeling good about ourselves is guilt. We grow prematurely old, put on excess weight, allow our bodies to deteriorate, turn away from sex, and deny our talents because we do not feel ourselves worthy of the pleasures and rewards of living a full life. Having judged ourselves guilty, we impose the most drastic of punishments: self-destruction.

At one time the distinction between right and wrong was sharply delineated. You committed a sin for which you would be punished in an afterlife. But if you confessed that sin, the burden of guilt was lifted. It was all beautifully simple.

In these enlightened times we are more tolerant of transgressions of the moral code and indeed often experience difficulty in determining what is right and what is wrong. While this attitude is certainly more civilized in that it permits each of us to lead our own lives within broad latitudes of acceptance, it has the big defect of throwing the burden of guilt squarely on the individual. For despite three-quarters of a century of psychoanalysis, we still have not eradicated the destructive effects of guilt. We have merely removed from everyday life the place where we can find absolution.

To keep guilt feelings from getting out of control, we must learn to accept all of ourselves and to see our lives in the broad perspective of humanity where no one of us is perfect.

Your Positive Profile

No one excells in everything; everyone excells in something.

To conquer feelings of guilt, inadequacy, and inferiority, draw a positive profile of yourself. Start now by listing on a sheet of paper all the things you do well. It might be driving a car, typing, speaking a foreign language, playing golf, embroidering, dancing, decorating, investing, gardening, performing your job. Write down whatever comes to mind. Experience confirms that you can perform these activities as well as anyone.

Now list your past achievements. This may require a little more introspection because we often downgrade as taken-for-granted inconsequentialities what are in reality important accomplishments. So be careful not to shortchange yourself. Overcoming an inclination to laziness in getting to work on time each morning is a definite accomplishment. Making plants grow in poor soil is an achievement. Maintaining one's cheerfulness and equilibrium in a trying family or job situation is noteworthy.

Now list your physical assets: eyes, bone structure, hair, complexion, figure, dimples, muxcles, flat abdomen, nicely shaped legs, etc.

And then your positive attitudes, which may be cheerfulness, fortitude, courage, curiosity, kindness, sympathy, patience. Again, these attributes may have become so integral a part of your personality that you do not credit them to yourself. "But that's just the way I am," you say, refusing to acknowledge the true worth of these characteristics.

I have a friend who repeatedly berates herself for being such a poor conversationalist. Nevertheless, others relish talking to her because she is such a sympathetic listener. When I pointed out that this was a gift of which she should be proud, she protested, "But I'm so dull, I can rarely think of what to say."

Finally, list the grow-young activities in which you are involved as a result of reading this book. "How can I credit to myself these actions that I am just beginning?" you may ask. Because starting actions to grow young is an achievement in itself. It signals a determination to master your existence and to live joyously and to the fullest extent possible. Don't underestimate the significance of beginnings.

In the very act of drawing up this "positive profile," you will have done much to conquer the feelings of guilt and inadequacy that haunt all of us from time to time. There are many reasons for feeling good about yourself.

A Short Guide to Thinking Better of Yourself

Accept your negative emotions—whether they be fear, anger, jealousy, hostility—as part of the human condition. Whenever the distorting mirror reflects them back to you larger than life-size, look to the other emotions listed in your "positive profile." You will see that you also have a great capacity for kindness, sympathy, courage, and love.

Place failure in perspective. Behind every successful invention stretches a long history of attempts at success that never came off. Look upon life as a continuous series of probings rather than as a giant test that you either pass or fail. As a noted writer once said, "the journey, not the arrival, matters."

Live in the present. The efforts you make today can change your life tomorrow. What is past you cannot change. Too often we waste our days brooding over an act committed years ago, accumulating a burden of guilt that drains our energy and makes us old long before our time. What's done is done. The future lies before you.

Frightened as children, some of us never lose our fear of the dark or of certain animals. Told by parents in a moment of anger that we are "stupid" or "ugly," we sometimes live with this negative profile for the rest of our days. All right! So that's what they said—and they were wrong. They had their own problems and pressures, and instead of dealing with them positively, they just unloaded them onto a scapegoat—you. But that's no excuse for continuing the assault on your personality. Because you do know better. Your "positive profile'' yields all kinds of instances proving the blanket indictment to be wrong. Now is the time to set the record straight—and accept yourself.

Don't try to be a paragon of all the virtues. There are occasions when anger clears the air, jealousy clarifies your feelings for another, and fear can save your life. It's a healthy practice to analyze the occasion for your emotion and to keep it in control. But don't try to live up to some impossibly high standard of conduct.

We all get into situations in which others need to feel superior to us and seek reassurance by putting us down. Recognize this for what it *is*: a cry for help and not a personal attack on yourself. Draw on your reserve of sympathy and understanding and give them the reassurance they so desperately need. They will soon stop criticizing.

Realize that comparisons are misleading and based on distorted images. We look at another person with attributes that we lack and think, ''If only . . .'' Yet if we knew the reality of the other's life, we would not change places with him for the world.

You enter a room full of the ''beautiful people.'' Everyone turns to you in admiration, your talents, virtues, intelligence immediately apparent. End of television commercial. . . . Now let us try a more realistic scene—and a more satsifying one. You enter a room, and no one immediately notices your presence. They are too self-absorbed or engrossed with others. You are neither crushed nor put down. Confident of your own worth, feeling good about yourself, accepting your uniqueness, you do not depend on the exaggerated acclaim of others for a verification of ''you.'' In the social situation you discern possibilities for conversation, for observation, perhaps making a new friend. And that is enough. Knowing who you are, you concentrate on enjoyment.

Give yourself a chance. All of us suffer from ''off days'' when our energy touches bottom. That's when feelings of guilt and inferiority seem to rush in, warping our better judgment and blurring from view the values of our ''positive profile.'' Admit that this is a bad day. Pamper yourself. Postpone critical tasks. And look forward to tomorrow.

Tapping Your Energy Resources

Have you ever remarked admiringly on some handsome and vigorous sixty-year old and wondered, "Where does he (or she) get all that youthful energy?"

The answer is, from the same internal fountain of youth shared by everyone. All of us possess energy resources that we fail to tap to their fullest extent.

"The human individual lives far within his limits," wrote William James, the noted American psychologist. Our organism has "deeper and deeper strata of explosible material, ready for use by anyone who probes so deep."

Then why do we so often hold back, settling for so little when we can have so much?

Mostly it is because we do not recognize the existence of these resources, bypassing with a taken-for-granted glance forces that could change our lives.

Sometimes it is because of a mistaken belief that we can hoard our energy, store it away for "later on." But that is like giving up walking or indeed any kind of exercise so that by age seventy we will have conserved sufficient muscle power to turn professional athlete. Of course it is quite the opposite that happens. The more we use our energy, the more freely it flows through our lives.

Now let us look at some of the energy resources available to each of us:

Confidence

Whatever you do well becomes a source of energy, whether it be your job, repairing a car, baking a cake, playing golf or tennis, collecting antiques or sewing. Fix these achievements firmly and proudly in your mind. Don't just take them for granted. Whenever you get depressed because of some situation that appears to be more than you can handle, switch your mind over to your proven skills and accomplishments. Let confidence unlock your energy.

Love

Do something for others: a word or gesture that dispels their loneliness or brings a moment of brightness into their lives; an offer of help where it is needed; in some way, give of yourself. Unselfish love takes you deep within yourself, where lie the sources of youthful energy.

Goals

Set yourself a goal and then push yourself to achieve it. You will discover that with sufficient motivation you can work many hours without fatigue, accomplish things you always thought outside your limits, for goals are among the most important energizers.

Mind Flexing

Acquire new ideas, invite change. Instead of immediately saying, "No," when someone suggests a work or play project that runs counter to your life style, say, "Why not?" Listen, investigate, ask questions, and try to be honest with yourself. Should you give it a try? What have you got to lose?

Taking a positive and youthful attitude toward the new and untried causes you to repeatedly tap your energy sources anew and to strain psychologically to comprehend new realms of experience. And the more new interests you build into your life, the more channels for the release of your energy you open up.

Conditioning

Each day, condition your mind and body to fuller energy use. Do a little more than the occasion calls for. Walk a little farther than is customary, take three exercise breaks instead of two.

Even if you don't feel like it, stand up at the town meeting and make yourself heard. Visit an acquaintance who is hospitalized, start on that cleaning or repair project you have been postponing. Get into the habit of tapping your resources for an increasingly bigger supply of energy. Expect more energy—and you will find more.

Friends

React to others. Share their excitement or pleasure. Voice your opinion. Experience the sheer "otherness" of friends and acquaintances. Observe them as if for the first time. Admit to yourself that you feel desire, antipathy, or whatever emotion they arouse in you. Come away from a meeting with another richer in mind and spirit. Discard your shield of indifference and allow others to energize you.

Peace of Mind

For at least half an hour each day, try to banish distraction, agitation, petty annoyances from your mind. Travel inward alone to the source of joy and renewal. Once more clear the channels of the daily accumulation of impediments that block the flow of your energy. (See the chapter, "A Time For Quiet.")

Sensuous Pleasures

Experience the sensuous world: the sounds of the city between midnight and daybreak; the smell of roasting coffee—or of the countryside after a spring rain; the taste of fresh fruit or of an exotic sauce; the sight of tall buildings outlined against the sunset or of a tiny garden in bloom; the touch of fabrics, of carved forms, of a body you love.

The senses refresh, restore, revitalize. Through the senses you find your way back to the primal world, re-establish the connections that get tangled and broken amid the bustle of everyday living.

Rewards

As you increasingly tap your energy resources, reward yourself along the way. If you walk an extra mile or work an hour longer, treat yourself at the end to some small indulgence. Associate energy use with pleasure, the good things of life.

Interests

Tap an interest and you tap an energy resource. You may say after a day of routine work, "I don't have an ounce of energy left." But develop a strong interest in sports, gardening, collecting, local politics, and watch the change.

Suddenly you have tapped a new energy source. Tiredness slips from you. And for one or more hours you are buoyantly living as though fatigue were something you never experienced. The long-term interest or hobby that recharges you over and over again is the most effective, for it enables you to switch from "boredom" or "weariness" to "energy" almost at will.

Obligations

Turn obligatory and unpleasant tasks into energizers. We all face them—dreary work that just has to be done, confrontations we would do anything to avoid, deadlines we keep moving ahead and ahead.

Avoided or allowed to drift, they build into crises. But face up to these situations, plan intelligently how to handle them, and you experience a tremendous rush of exhilaration. You feel ready for anything now. The moral is clear: Each time you tap your energy sources with confidence, you emerge with a new realization of your powers.

The Past

You would not be alive and reading this book unless you had learned to tap at least some of your energy resources. And if you look back on the time when you conquered an illness, lived through a bad time, completed a miserable task, managed to fight an uphill battle to get through school or to hold your family together, went out of your way to help a friend, you will realize that, without thinking about it, you tapped far more resources that you would customarily use.

That you could automatically perform so many energy-demanding actions over a period of time should give you some idea of the powers at your disposal.

Momentum

"Get going"—and you gather momentum. Push yourself to your outer limits in one activity and you gain additional energy for others. Work at your exercise program consistently and you make it easier to develop good eating habits. Impose discipline on the way you maintain your clothes and you are more likely to improve your posture. Develop your skill in sports or crafts or macrame and your ability to undertake other projects grows. Every additional activity adds to your self-confidence. Energy thrives on use.

Fun

Fun is doing something for the sheer enjoyment of it. It may be climbing a mountain, putting up strawberry preserves, dancing, walking through the city in search of throwaway treasures, dressing up for dinner with a few friends, or spending an evening listening to records that were popular when we were teen-agers.

Whatever it may be, fun triggers a spontaneous release of energy that sends us back to our serious purposes revitalized and recharged. Now the advice to have fun may appear redundant in the seventies, but the frantic competitiveness and desperation that underlie so many of the activities that are misnamed fun today do more to wear us out than energize us. So discover your own meaning of fun—and then let go.

Nature

Go swimming. Walk through the countryside—and bring your lunch along. Lie on the grass and observe the sunlight filtering through the leaves of the trees. Listen—really listen—to the sound of a brook, the distant hoot of a train whistle. And spend at least part of the time alone. Stop for the night at a small inn or hotel off the beaten path and rise with the dawn.

Beauty

Visit the museums and art galleries. Look at the paintings and sculpture without bothering to check them in the catalogue. You can get the facts another time. Today, just react, enjoy, see. Return again to those works that please and intrigue you. Make them part of your own mental collection, your "museum without walls."

Don't give up after the first visit, Go back several times until art becomes a natural part of your life, a source on which you can draw in moments of contemplation.

Religion

Over the centuries man has looked to belief in some superior being, some idea of order above the chaos of the universe, for strength, consolation, and energy. For some, religion has meant churches, creeds, a life lived according to specific disciplines. For others, it has meant a personal relationship with the divine spirit. Either way, the search for some transcendental "connection" will open to you a source of power to sustain you for the duration of your days.

Get Going: Nineteen Grow-Young Action Projects

Get involved and grow young; or remain on the sidelines while life rushes by: That's the alternative we all face.

Fortunately, we live in an age when opportunities for creative and revitalizing involvement abound.

Whatever our background, economic status, job, or age, we can participate in projects that will make us look and feel younger while enriching our lives.

Instead of inventing excuses why we can't get involved, let us concentrate our thoughts on discovering ways in which we can.

Select two from among the nineteen grow-young action projects listed below and take the plunge—now. Better yet, explore a few of them in succession. And give each a fair chance to turn you on before you turn it off. Even from those that turn out to be not exactly your cup of tea you will come away with a broader perspective on the opportunities open to you and the kind of uplift that comes from any new experience.

To grow young, get going!

Community Participation

Take some responsibility for making your community a better place. Planting trees or flowers, day-care centers, food for the needy, getting out the vote, helping on committees to aid the disabled, are just a few of the areas in which men and women of all ages involve themselves in responsible activism.

Any one can become a citizen activist. All you need is a desire to work with others to improve local conditions.

Select some area about which you feel strongly and then search out some group that is working for change. Your local newspaper can assist you in making contacts.

But perhaps no group yet exists for the job you believe worth doing—maybe it is to save some historic building from demolition or to prevent a superhighway from bulldozing its way through your neighborhood. In that case, start your own campaign. Talk about the need for action to everyone you meet and insert a small and inexpensive classified ad in your local newspaper. "Anyone interested in saving Jones Street contact XYZ."

When the letters and phone calls start coming in, set a date for a meeting at your place, the local library, or town hall. And you are on your way.

The great thing about community action is the way it brings together people of diverse backgrounds. Galvanized by a common cause, strangers swiftly become friends. The individual with no exciting goals or interest overnight turns into a person full of purpose, excitement, and energy.

Involved, committeed, connecting with others, we inevitably feel younger, think younger, act younger, and look younger.

Collect

Join that delightful and ageless elite, the collectors. Collectors of what?

Of antiques, art, books, bottles, cameos, china, fabrics, documents, embroidery, farm implements, records, shells, silverware—you name it.

Continuously fascinated by the chase, searching everywhere for some clue that will lead to the discovery of one more item to add to "the collection," the true collector possesses neither the time nor the patience for boredom and premature aging.

Few people have bridged the generation gap so successfully as those with a passion for collectiong, At any gathering you will observe long-haired teen-agers and grandparents avidly exchanging gossip and arranging the swap of items that each believes will reinforce the prestige of his or her collection.

How do you start collecting?

Consult a few of the books in your library on any of the categories suggested above—or any others you find in the hobby section. Browse among these volumes until you discover a subject that arouses your curiosity. Location, too, may play a part in your selection. Gathering seashells does not come easily to inland dwellers, but city streets offer rich provender in the way of old furniture, pictures, prints, and other discarded items that may turn out to be real treasures.

Once you have chosen your specialty, start reading everything you can find about it. The classified ads in the papers offer many leads for swaps and deals. Pursue the chase into antique shops and secondhand stores, ask your friends about the "junk" hidden in their attics, and don't be too proud to poke around when "trash" is being thrown out. Some collectors gleefully return from these scavenging expeditions with truly valuable "finds."

Talk to the people at the shops about your interest. Often they can put you in touch with fellow enthusiasts. When you want to exchange an item, take out a tiny ad in one of the specialized newspapers or magazines. This, too, will open doors to your ever-widening circle of collector friends.

Stay on the alert for special exhibitions, auctions,

meetings, and make a point of attending a few. You will meet more people—and also get an opportunity to "Keep up with the market." You may not want to sell what you have collected, but it is great fun to learn that similar items are fetching high prices.

As a collector, you never lack for conversational material. And soon you will discover that friends and strangers will be calling on you for "an opinion" on something they found in a shop or have inherited from Aunt Hattie.

Many a true collector finds his greatest delight in getting something for nothing—or almost. It is no sport to spend lavishly. Indeed, when collectors gather, the proudest boast is how little something cost, not that it was expensive.

Collecting is far more than acquisitiveness. It is high adventure. No wonder so many collectors retain their youthful vigor throughout the years.

Theater

Get into the act!

Be a director, playwright, actor or actress, costume or set designer, lighting technician, publicity manager. Whatever your age, amateur theater has a place for you.

Here is an opportunity to enter a fascinating world in which background and experience count for little. On the stage, the student, secretary, clerk, doctor, housewife, assembly-line worker, bus driver, writer, shed their workaday identities to assume the roles written by Shakespeare, Ibsen, Chekhov, Shaw, and Beckett.

With millions of us focused on our television sets, we tend to lose sight of the increasing dramatic activities of little theater groups, churches, schools, and community art councils. Yet today there exist few areas in which small groups are not busily at work rehearsing an upcoming theatrical treat for their neighbors.

Look for announcements in the newspapers, inquire at churches and libraries, and as soon as you discover news of a forthcoming production, contact the sponsors. Spell out your interests, which may range from acting to carpentering and sewing. (Someone has to make those sets and costumes.)

Don't let shyness hold you back. Once on stage with the group, you inhabit a world in which everyone supports everyone else. The current flows, and you come alive in a new way.

Crafts

Be creative. Make something.

Some of the happiest and most youthful people in the world today are the craftsmen and craftswomen. It is easy to see why. With just a few inexpensive tools and materials and a few feet of work space, they are nevertheless privileged to join the eminent company of "makers" whose work has come down to us across the ages. Whether world-famous like Benvenuto Cellini or anonymous like the woodcarvers whose statues grace the medieval cathedrals, the craftsman is continuously revitalized by having at hand some bit of work that demands his skill and attention.

Discover a craft that interests you—and you have discovered the perfect antidote for worry, depression, nervousness, boredom, and premature age. Both those of us who work at monotonous tasks and those who work under mental tension can be sure of finding refreshment and renewal when we turn to our workbench for an hour or two.

But crafts offer more than therapy. They yield a sense of achievement and aesthetic satisfaction in our handiwork. What's more, we can frequently turn our skills into moneymaking opportunities, even small businesses. Much of the public has become fed up with cheap imitation "crafts" objects made by machine and is searching for the "real thing," so that it may be possible to market your creations through local merchants or sell them directly from your home by advertising in selected journals and newspapers.

Craftsmen, like collectors, tend to be a passionate breed. They like nothing better than to exchange notes about their projects, tools and materials, and will travel many miles to attend an exhibition.

As with collecting, start with your library or bookstore and spend an hour or two browsing among books on woodworking, enameling, sewing crafts, leathercrafting, silversmithing, cabinetmaking, etc. Some of the manufacturers of tools and materials offer free catalogues that can prove useful in estimating the space and cost requirements of your craft. A word of caution: Don't go overboard on purchasing costly tools. Start with the bare minimum and work your way up.

Bicycling

Get a bike and see the world. You see precious little of it in a jet or driving along a superhighway. But pedal through a deserted city street or country lane and once again the world takes on a human aspect. There is time to look at buildings and flowers and to stop and investigate a shop or a patch of woods when the mood suits you.

Biking is one of the all-around grow-young activities. While on two wheels you can enjoy healthful exercise, sociability, history, culture, exploration, and travel. You can join dedicated groups of bikers who visit nothing but churches and cathedrals. Others explore the city from midnight to dawn.

Walking Tours

Join or organize a walking tour. Every weekend in cities and towns you will discover small groups pouring over maps and peering interestedly at old buildings or ruins before they move on to their next destination. Strangers when they started out, these walkers with a purpose soon become friends as they explore a particular segment of the world.

Walking tours afford a singularly human form of activity in our mechanized society. In the cities you discover how people live and work on those streets beneath which the subway hurtles you to and from the job. In the country you learn the meaning that distance held for our premotorized ancestors.

Walking tours can be organized with as few as three and as many as fifteen people. Any more tends to get unwieldly. The occasions for the tour can be as varied as your interests: historical tours, literary tours, collectors' tours, tree tours, barn tours, painting, wild flower and garden tours.

Start with a street or area map, draw an itinerary originating at some mutually convenient point, and trace a line from one location to another, If you are organizing the tour, read up on the subject and make notes on separate cards, giving as much information as possible about the places you plan to visit.

A good way to build maximum participation is to ask each member of the tour to research a different book or source—so that everyone contributes to the general store of information.

If you don't know people who might want to join, place a classified ad in the local newspaper or tack a notice to the bulletin board at your shopping center or place of business.

Explore Nature

Spend a day in the country collecting wildflowers and

exotic ferns. An inexpensive illustrated paperback will help identify the various species and open up a new world. Words like Lady slipper and verbascum will start to roll off your tongue as authoritatively as if you were a horticulturist. Soon, wherever you walk, in the city or countryside, peering into gardens and yards, you will find yourself among friends.

Or go fishing. No other sport offers this unique combination of breathless excitement and contemplative peace. To see what a truly happy individual looks like, observe an angler in early May waiting for the first bite.

Watch the birds, alone or with a bird-watching group. These amateur ornithologists will often rise before dawn and gather in some field or city park on the chance that they will see some rare bird in migration. Here is a fine way to attune your senses to the natural world that still exists beneath the ubiquitous clamor and clutter of present-day technology.

Flowers, birds, fish, clear streams, and open fields need every friend they can find to save them from the depredations of "progress." So why not combine your interest in nature with an active defense of these precious resources? Join one of the ecological groups operating near you, or organize one. Volunteer your services and do your bit to keep nature from sinking into premature age.

Travel

Plan a trip to some place that has always fascinated you. Or just collect travel folders and browse through them until you respond. Once you have fixed your destination, read everything about it you can lay your hands on. New travel books—and history books published a century ago. Dip into some of the region's literature, brush up on native dishes, handicrafts, customs. Immerse yourself.

Then explore alternate routes and budgets. Search for out-of-the-way places to stay. Write directly to the hotels and try to elicit from a recent visitor a few tips gleaned from his experience.

You may spend only two weeks and comparatively little money on the actual trip, but the fun you have doing the research and the planning and the knowledge you bring to the sites will make it seem ever so much longer.

Go Back to School

Acquire a foreign language. Discover what the "new novel" is all about. Learn to operate a small printing press in your basement. Explore the thoughts of the ancient philosophers.

But there just isn't space to list the adult-education courses available today. Send for the catalogues of all schools within commuting distance and make your selection. Don't hesitate because of fears that your mind may have grown too "rusty" or because of unpleasant memories of grades and exams. All you need to qualify in the open world of modern adult education is curiosity. And don't deny yourself the pleasure of experiencing new ideas, new friends, and indeed a new life because you work hard during the day and have no energy left for anything by evening. Once you start feeling the exhilaration that springs from involvement in a subject that interests you, that tiredness will drop away and you will marvel at your renewed energy.

Learning is one of the basic grow-young activities. It can transform you mentally and physically. Get into it now.

Exploration

Set out for nowhere. With an empty afternoon or evening before you, take a bus you never rode before—to the end of the line. Or get off the train in a strange town and just walk around. If you live in the city, spend a day in the country (and vice versa). Relish the change of scene, the different pace, the possibilities of another kind of life. What would your existence be like if . . . ?

The Past Revisited

Contact someone you have not seen for years. The experience may shake you up a bit, but it will also deepen your capacity for sympathy and understanding. Observing how others have changed can jolt us out of our lethargy and spark major change in our lives.

Grow Young with Youth

Spend time with young people. Listen, participate, enjoy. Open yourself to their rhythms, attitudes, styles. And give of yourself.

Explore the shops featuring the styles of the young designers. Subscribe to one of the youth-culture papers. When traveling, dining out, serving on committees, talk to young people. Ask questions, make an attempt to understand what they are really saying and don't patronize. Best of all, make some teen-age friends. Common interests—biking, collecting, sports, music—all serve to break down the artificial generation barriers and restore us to our common humanity.

Ask for Help

If you don't know what to do about your job, if you have an emotional problem you can't handle, if you don't know how to color-coordinate your clothes, call up someone you know and explain the problem. Frankly admit, "I need help," and ask, "Do you have a few minutes to listen?" Nine times out of ten, the other will not only be sympathetic but flattered. Even if the advice proves unusable, just talking about the problem helps put it into perspective.

Organize an Event

It might be getting a few neighbors together to discuss a community project; taking a few children to a museum or for a walk in the woods; opening your home for a charity sale; teaching youngsters to play tennis, knit, or carve; or planning a workshop in which jazz enthusiasts or classical music buffs can listen to records, tape radio concerts, criticize performances, and plan local record festivals.

Live Without Money

Do completely without money for a day. Walk to work, take your lunch, search out free entertainment, skip the newspapers, make no telephone calls, turn off the television and radio, sup by the light of a candle.

Experience Your Body

Close the door behind you, take off all your clothes, and live naked for an evening. Take a long, relaxing bath, move rhythmically to music, read, watch television, lie stretched out on the bed, sew—all in the buff, climate permitting!

Plan

Plan a vacation, a reading program, a new career. Plan to redecorate your room, to cultivate a garden, to lose ten pounds. Plan to start a diary, to acquire a new skill. Push outward the limits of what you have heretofore considered possible.

Change Your Plumage

Try a new wardrobe. (You don't have to buy it.) Spend a day in the shops examining and trying on the kind of clothes you don't usually purchase. Ask the sales people for suggestions. Experiment with unusual color combinations. Forget about prices. You can always find less expensive equivalents. Don't buy on this trip. Just come away with ideas, new horizons for your personal style.

Start Something

The world is full of people waiting for the telephone to ring. Dial someone who may be alone and invite them over for tea, a drink, dinner. Suggest a movie or a walk. And don't be snobbish about age. Teen-agers and older people get lonely, too—and you may be surprised at what they have to contribute.

Wherever you live, you will find opportunities for involvement. Search them out. Explore as many as you can. Experiment. But get moving now. Step out from the sidelines and into the mainstream. Plan to begin at least one grow-young action project today.

The Magic of Change

Would you like to look and feel twenty years younger?

Then make a change in your life.

A change of job, a move to a different neighborhood, the discovery of a new life style, can trigger a profound release of youthful energy and snap the chain of tensions and frustrations that has been holding you down.

Doctors tell of patients whose inexplicable headaches suddenly disappear when they change their work or environment. The executive and the housewife who complain of chronic fatigue are discovered to be tired of just one thing—the old routine.

Fortunately, we live in an age when the magic of change lies within reach of most of us. Each year, some thirty-six million Americans change residence, mostly in pursuit of different jobs and different life styles "elsewhere." Add to them the growing number of on-the-go-ers in Britain and in Europe and the proportion of the West's population enamored of change is impressive indeed.

Just a decade ago, job-switching was frowned upon. Mergers, acquisitions, technology, the cultural swing away from security and toward a fuller life, have now made job-changing the accepted life style of millions.

In the words of Professor Harry Levinson of the Harvard Business

School, it is now permissible "to think of alternatives . . . It has become quite legitimate to have freedom of choice, to be fresh, to use one's talents better."

It's not just executives who believe that life begins anew with a second career. According to one recent survey, "middle-aged housewives have become the most aggressive career switchers in the past decade," flooding back into the business world in search of personal income, a challenging job, and the chance to meet new people and once more get involved with life's mainstream.

"What—Change Jobs at My Age?"

> A Philadelphia department-store executive suffered from ulcers, could not break the worry habit, and was fast sinking into premature age. He chucked it all and became a policeman in a small town. He liked his new work so much that he stayed on even after his ulcers were cured.
>
> A schoolteacher in Buffalo, frustrated and bitter with the red tape of the educational system and the lack of satisfaction in his work, moved with his wife and four children to an Indian reservation in Arizona where he is now happy in his new teaching job.
>
> A Detroit assembly-line worker with twenty years seniority quit his secure job, sold his home in the suburbs, and gambled all to open a fishing camp in the Minnesota lake country.
>
> A chemical company arbitration executive, bypassed for advancement by a twenty-six-year-old "whiz kid," quit in dudgeon. He became a tennis "pro" in a small resort town and reports he has "never felt younger in my life."
>
> A veteran saleslady in a London department store quit after fifteen years on the job and moved to a small city where she

invested her savings to become part owner in a dress shop. The air is cleaner, the pace is slower, and she enjoys the kind of friendly atmosphere of which she had always dreamed.

A thirty-eight-year-old secretary began attending evening school out of boredom. She became interested in engineering ecology and is now on the way to becoming a specialist in that field.

"Getting fired is the best thing that happened to me," reports an electronics engineer. He took a "desperation" job with a building reclamation contractor and now gets immense personal satisfaction out of helping to save nineteenth-century buildings from the wrecker's ball.

An Atlanta housewife, caught up in community work to improve the local school system, found the job so fascinating that she is studying nights and plans to run for office.

A couple in their mid-forties, fed up with almost two decades of big-city clerical work and with little to show for it, took to the road as "Mr. and Mrs. Fix-It."

Deciding to Change

Obviously, change is possible.

Then why do we sometimes hold back? Never even get started?

Because with family, financial, educational, or whatever other considerations may be involved, change seems like such a long-range proposition.

Yet it really isn't.

We begin to reap the rewards of job-changing the moment we make up our minds to change.

The frustrations, tensions, anxieties associated with the old job, begin to lift when we introduce the prospect of major change into our lives.

As long as we can see no way out of our predicament, with vistas of nothing but more of the same stretching before us, we are wide open to psychological fatigue and premature aging.

Given the realistic hope for change—hope that is buttressed by planning, preparation, action—we walk with a new buoyancy and action.

The decision to change marks a big step forward on the path to growing young.

Dreaming and Doing

The more we dream of changing our job, the more likely we are to make the change.

Dreams sustain us during low periods and repeatedly recharge our motivational batteries.

So don't be afraid to fantasize a bit about the change you want to make. This is your way of familiarizing yourself with the strange territory ahead. And increasingly, you will find that your dreams take place in a practical frame of reference. You will find yourself trying to particularize, to pin down the place and the job and what life will be like.

From dreaming to doing then becomes a short step. Sift your dreams to arrive at your real interests—those that have stayed with you over the years and that recur again and again. They may be as general as working out of doors, or owning a small business. They may be as specific as teaching, opening a small crafts shop in a resort town, or getting secretarial work in a publisher's office. Try to separate the mere whim from the abiding interest.

Then check your "resources," present and potential, for entering your chosen field. Isolate the things (1) you like to do and (2) can do well—or could with the right training. When they coincide, you are on the right track to successful change.

Get all the information you can about your chosen field. Talk to people in the business. Sound out acquaintances who have some experience in the field. This kind of "inside info" can add immeasurably to the success of your job change.

Read everything you can lay your hands on that touches on your interest. Discover where you might fit in, what training might be required, and where to get it.

Then set your campaign rolling. Start with friends, asking for leads and suggestions. Begin a letter-writing campaign to prospective employers. The more people you write and talk to, the more "advertisers" there are working for you.

Holding on to your present job "in the meanwhile" can take the economic pressure off the search for change. It's also a good idea to start a little "second career" savings account to cushion the transition.

Don't postpone enjoying your big decision to change until the day you actually walk out of your job. Reap some of the grow-young rewards now.

You have taken the big step of deciding, which has given you a new perspective on life. You are no longer "standing still" while the world goes by but moving under your own power in a new and youthful direction. You may even find some aspects of your present job enjoyable, now that you have set off in the direction of change.

Learning to Change

Going back to school may seem like a roundabout way of bringing major change into our lives, but it isn't. We may start out with a desire to expand the dimensions of our personal world—to share in the wonderful discoveries of science, pick up the threads of history or philosophy that were severed by family responsibilities or the need to earn a living, or develop our talents as "Sunday painters." But soon we find that our few hours in evening class are breaking down the barriers of habit that hem us in and obscure the possibilities of change. We make new friends, gain the self-confidence that comes from being "with it" instead of on the sidelines.

While learning and enjoying the contact with different people and ideas, we are acquiring the courage to redirect our lives. From our new vantage point, changing jobs or moving to another city no longer looms so formidably. Through action, we acquire a fresh perspective on what is possible.

In acquiring confidence in our ability to accept new ideas, to learn new ways of thinking and acting, to mingle with people of different backgrounds and interests, we also gain the confidence necessary to grow into a new and youthful life style.

Use Your Interests as a Springboard for Change

If you want to see a man or woman glowing with youthful vitality, look for the person with active interests. The gardener, for example, is continuously involved with tomorrow—with the new buds springing to life, with the soil that needs to be worked for next year's flower bed, with getting the right mixture of sun and shade for the blooms that will beautify the back yard—or the apartment window box. When gardeners meet—in the office or on the way to work—they bubble with enthusiasm, never at a loss for conversation. In their world, something is always happening, and change is the order of the day.

Now few of us are born gardeners—or railroad buffs, amateur chefs, linguists, antique collectors, or whatever. Mostly these activities are sparked by a decision to change one's life. The rewards of the job or the house in the suburbs or family life have not turned out quite as expected. But rather than acquiesce in the succession of little defeats that add up to profound dissatisfaction with one's lot, these amateurs have refreshed their life with the magic of change.

But that is not all. Many have used their interests as a springboard for a major change in their life styles, turning their hobbies into practical ventures. The person who knows that he or she can always "get along" by exercising their amateur skills in crafts or gardening or buying and selling old furniture is continuously reassured by the ability to manage change.

In the section on grow-young activities, I list many areas of amateur activity that may come to play important roles in your life. Build at least one or two of these into your program for change. They bring their own rewards in enjoyment and achievement, and throughout the years they enhance your options for change.

Don't Let Others Stop You: Strategies for Countering Criticism

"Act your age!"

You may as well start preparing right now to encounter some version of that put-down remark intended to shame or ridicule you into abandoning your grow-young program.

Especially at the beginning, one or more members of your family may flare up indignantly at what they consider to be your betrayal of an unsigned but binding agreement to bow down to premature age.

The wife notices her husband breaking out of his established routine. Instead of settling down before the television set each evening, he involves himself in community affairs and invites his new friends into the house for discussions about local politics. Or he begins passing up his favorite dessert, lets his hair grow a bit longer, and comes home with a tie several hues bolder than any he has worn in years.

Understandably, the wife is upset. She senses a threat to her security as defined by the established pattern of their life together. She may suspect that her husband, with his new interests, his trimmer figure, and get-up-and-go energy may be moving on and leaving her behind. Maybe another woman is involved. In self-defense, she turns the full force of her scorn and ridicule on his efforts at self-renewal.

Then there's the husband suddenly confronted by this strange woman, the mother of his children, who insists on returning to school so she can brush up on her secretarial skills and go back to work. One afternoon she returns from downtown with a new hairdo and a book on yoga exercises. He realizes that his wife is changing, making an effort to grow more alert, attractive, and interesting. But instead of responding with encouragement, he feels threatened and voices his fear in terms of ridicule. "Act your age," he blurts out.

Teen-agers can be the most withering of all in their comments. Sometimes a glance is sufficient to express their scorn for a parent's grow-young program. At other times their protests, reinforced by appeals to "what will my friends think," can be deafening. For while youth believes it is just fine for their generation to overthrow the conventions, just let a parent deviate from what the youngsters consider prescribed conduct for anyone over thirty, and the howls of indignation never cease.

Turning Ridicule into Support

When members of the family ridicule your actions for change, they are really expressing their own insecurity. They may fear that in breaking out of the premature age bind, getting your body into shape, and developing new interests you are breaking the bonds that hold you together. Your rejection of the rich dessert, of the chair in front of the television set, of the around-the-clock housewife role, they interpret as a rejection of themselves.

Fearing that "the new you" will no longer love "the old them," they desperately try to hold you back from change. Defensively they strike out at grow-young activities with the first weapon that comes to hand: ridicule. "Act your age."

Once you grasp the reason for these attacks, it becomes easier to counter them. With a little determination and strategy, you can even turn this hostility into support.

Communicate

The key lies in communication. Now few of us are so persuasive and articulate that we can present to a skeptical family audience a comprehensive and glowing picture of our grow-young program and expect to win immediate, wholehearted support.

But we can convey the all-important assurance that our efforts to change do not spell a diminishing of our love—indeed, that we would like nothing better than to share our adventure.

Begin by talking in terms of shared concerns, for example. Express your determination to lose a few pounds through more sensible eating habits. This will more than justify changing the pattern of your meals.

Health also offers an acceptable explanation for a program of exercises, taking up new sports, walking to work, or joining a bicycling club. About practically any health-promoting activity you can remark to your family, "It makes me feel years younger. Why don't you try it with me?" Take the lead, and the next time you go for a brisk walk, invite another along. Make an effort to get this member of the family into the swing of the thing and try to convey some of your own sense of purpose and enjoyment.

Another way to gain acceptance for your program is to join in an activity that others enjoy. Maybe your children play baseball, tennis, golf. Pursue these sports—with the children or on your own. This is something they understand, and they can only be proud of your accomplishments.

It's How You Say It

Present your actions for change one at a time and in terms that relate to the other's interests. The housewife who is determined to change her life style by returning to work after years spent raising a family can expect little sympathy if she merely complains about being bored or having nothing to do all day. Thinking that he sure could use a little of that boring idleness himself, the hard-working husband turns an unsympathetic ear to what sounds like an unreasonable gripe.

But let the wife relate her plan to more income for the family, to an opportunity to take a trip or buy a new car, and chances are she will have created a favorable climate for change.

Innumerable ways exist to communicate assurance that your grow-young actions do not threaten the other. Instead of emerging from your room one day with a new wardrobe that contradicts your customary style of dressing, make the other a partner in your adventure. Plan a joint shopping expedition. Suggest that the other break out in a bit of extravagance and buy something different and daring. Help the other select some item that will contribute to a more youthful appearance—and express your admiration for the result. Then move on to your own purchase.

At home, encourage the wearing of new styles, not just on special occasions but every day. "But this is ridiculous," the other may protest at first. "Maybe it is," you reply. "But isn't it fun? And you must admit you look great."

It's not important that you share identical interests. You may enjoy gardening, the other golf. What is important is the help you give the other to discover equivalent grow-young interests.

But suppose you want to turn your life around, pull up stakes, quit your job, move from one part of the country to another? Again it is a "we" and not just a "me" proposition that calls for mutual exploration and discussion. If the change promises to give you freedom for growth and renewal but denies the needs of the other, you can be sure your freedom will prove illusionary. It is impossible to achieve a joyous and youthful existence at the expense of another.

Reassurance

You will remember that in the chapter on "Easy Starters" we talked about limbering up our attitudes and breaking the pattern of premature age. Here we are attempting to bring about a similar limbering up of the attitudes of others toward our grow-young actions, and that means reassuring them on two important points:

1. Our actions for change do not threaten their security or signal a falling off of our love;

2. We would be more than happy to share our adventure with them.

We communicate this reassurance by the manner in which we introduce our grow-young program—in terms of shared concerns such as health and a better life for the other as well as for ourselves. And we do it little by little. None of us are prepared for the shock of sudden change in a person whom we love. But we can guide them into the spirit of gradual change and thus build support for our efforts.

The Envy of Others

Married or single, you will inevitably find yourself in situations with friends and colleagues in which defending your grow-young actions will require as much strategy as within your own family.

If you have taken off a few pounds, they will wonder aloud if you have been ill. If you announce that you will be playing tennis tomorrow, they will turn overly solicitous about your heart. Walk into a room sporting a particularly colorful ascot or pair of slacks and you may be greeted by a sarcastic, "But aren't we being daring tonight."

Envy is never pleasant, and aggressive envy can sting, particularly when we are venturing something new that lacks the reinforcement of previous success. For a moment, we may be tempted to avoid the limelight and shrivel up in some corner rather than face another attack.

We may be tempted, but we do not succumb. For envy is the confirmation of our success. It marks the distance you have set between yourself and the others by your grow-young actions. That you should develop new interests, explore new life styles, use the full potential of your mind and body for joyous living, will always prove intolerable to the jealous ones.

Fortunately, the aggressively envious are in the majority. Their words can only hurt you if you permit them to deflect you from your course.

Whenever someone ridicules the activities of a grow-young friend of mine, she just smiles brightly and says, "But it's such fun. You should try it." And then goes on to another topic.

In short, stand your ground and others will soon stop badgering you.

Sometimes we see ridicule where none is intended. The first time we stride vigorously from home to the office instead of driving, the first time we enter a different restaurant alone and sporting a new hat, the first time we play a different sport, we self-consciously imagine that everyone is staring at us and wondering, "Whatever is this one up to?"

Actually, most people are too busy with their own preoccupations to give us more than a passing thought—if that much—to what we are up to. Seldom is the spotlight focused on ourselves.

But as you get involved in your grow-young program, you will occasionally notice strangers looking at you with sincere admiration. Friends will ask, "How do you do it?" And that's the time to be generous with the fruits of your experience and help others roll back the years and start living.

Springboards to a Youthful Appearance

Everything we do, not just our clothes and cosmetics, affects our appearance: our attitude toward ourselves and other people, how we spend our time, what we eat, the sleep we get, posture, exercise, and —especially—boredom. It's impossible to conceal ourselves from others.

Appearance is animation, the glint of an eye, the movements of hands and feet, the way the head is held. Action and reaction between the body and what it is wearing, the feel and appearance of confidence, hope or dejection, humor and sadness. The most fascinating faces are those that represent a person who has lived, in the fullest sense, and is proud of it and would not think of trying to conceal it. Joy, pain, dignity, guilt, fear, humor, dread, greed, love—these and many other emotions are expressed in our faces and in the way we carry our bodies.

What makes us *feel* good also makes us *look* good, and vice versa. The same elements make us feel and look youthful. Walking with head held high, a spring in the step and a feeling of optimism about ourselves says everything about us. A new hat, a jaunty scarf or gloves are as important for the effects they have on the wearer as on the person looking at them. Little things make such a difference, particularly if not taken too seriously.

Today there are many products and services available to help us improve our appearance. But first, it's important to realize that clothes and cosmetics, while important, can't do the whole job alone. Health, interesting things to do, love, projects to look forward to—these give us a lively, youthful look that no amount of beauty treatments can match in effectiveness. Armed with the ideas in this book and the determination to grow younger, you are bound to be successful.

For instant feel- and look-young results, take a deep breath, lift your chin, throw your head and shoulders back, pull your stomach in. Hold it a few seconds and then let go. Doesn't it feel great? With a small amount of time each day spent in changing a few aging habits, you'll soon be holding yourself erect without being conscious of the effort; you'll feel more rested and relaxed, more like doing all the things you've always dreamed of doing but haven't had quite enough confidence to attempt. Your slumping posture will be a thing of the past, and you'll be ready for a new suit to show off your new body. You'll soon be breathing more deeply, giving your heart and lungs more oxygen.

Remember that one success breeds another. There's nothing like it: Conquer one bad habit, achieve one degree of improvement, and you're off, ready to tackle another and another and another. It becomes easier with each achievement, and soon there will be nothing you won't attempt—not just in the way you look but in reaching for new goals in living.

One of the quickest ways to deposit a couple of successes in your confidence bank is through the way you look. This book offers a few suggestions; you'll think of others as you go along, suited to your own specific needs and goals.

Responding to People

Why talk about relating to people under appearance?

Think of the people you see who look youthful. Chances are that the ones who come to mind first are not necessarily handsome or beautiful in the movie star sense but in the alive way they react and respond to the people around them. They are not passive, never expressing their emotions and thoughts. They respond to the situation and the person of the moment, they are busy listening and reacting so that they literally don't have time to fidget and be self-conscious about their own appearance. These are the people who don't worry about wrinkles, gray hair, or other symptons of aging; they are too busy living and doing—and not always in complete happiness. Whether they are eighteen or eighty, we are not so much aware of their age as we are of them as individuals whose lives are full. Involvement, responsiveness, and continuing interest in the world around you, these will change the way you look.

Find Your Style

Should you try to imitate teen-agers or wear the "latest thing," whatever it is? More than likely, you'll feel better about the way you look if you avoid extremes. This sounds wishy-washy, but women should aim for softness without vagueness, clarity without hardness. Try to find your own style in the way you wear your hair, make-up and clothes. Be very selective in your buying from among the many tempting new fashions urged on you. Keep up with fashion but to the degree that suits you. Certainly you can't have a grow-young appearance without adopting some of the latest trends, but you don't want to look as if you're competing with teen-agers, either.

Sometimes changing apparance can make one feel a bit uncomfortable and conspicuous at first. Some people prefer to get used to something new by wearing it privately a few times before venturing to expose it to others. Some find it easier to plunge in. Let "them" be shocked if they want to be, but you're enjoying their reactions—and yourself—and it's quite likely they envy your courage. Changing one's appearance is fun—for you and for your family and friends, if done in the spirit of fun.

Reminder

Other chapters in this book deal with exercise, health, food, and keeping up to date in mind and spirit. Many of us have forgotten what we were taught about health and hygiene and nutrition and the importance of exercise. They are even more important now than they were when we were in school, so be sure to refresh your memory by reading those chapters. Your youthful appearance depends on it.

Special Note

You can learn about hair styling and make-up techniques and products from a few visits to a beauty salon. The specialists can help keep you from making expensive mistakes. It's true that some of them will try to sell you a whole array of make-up and beauty aids, but be selective and state honestly that you want to look younger and prettier but that you don't want items that unnecessarily complicate your good looks routine. If you enjoy spending a long time on making up, then do, but if you are not accustomed to doing this, you want something that will not be a chore. That would only defeat your purpose, you would soon abandon the project and feel defeated and old looking all over again. Be honest about this—don't invest in products that you're unlikely to use.

Hair

Male or female, one of the quickest ways to give your appearance an uplift is by a change of hair style. The shape and bearing of your head and facial features can all be made to look younger by the way you wear your hair.

Consider a Wig

> You can try on wigs or toupees in a salon or department store. This gives you an opportunity to see how you look with hair of a different length, different color or styling. You can then either buy the wig or toupee—or go to a stylist and have them duplicate the effect you found most pleasing. Some wigs are very inexpensive, especially those made of

man-made fibers. Human hair wigs cost more. Most wigs can be restyled and the color changed. The odds are against your being satisfied with a wig ordered by mail, so keep trying them on until you find one that is right for you. Custom-made wigs are naturally more expensive. More and more men and women are wearing them. Whether or not you buy one, don't overlook this as an easy way to experiment on how you want to change your hair style or color.

Which Hair Style for You?

As just mentioned, you might like to try a wig to find the answer to this question. Men will probably find that longer hair makes them look youthful, while women will find the opposite. To counteract the lines of aging in the face, you don't want the sagging, downward lines of long hair. Extra long hair usually starts looking bedraggled a day or two after a shampoo. Loosely curled hair makes the face look softer and more gentle—and younger—than severely straight hair. Give your face a chance to look its best; your hair is the "setting" or frame for it. And don't think that you're stuck with a style forever. Changing hair styles is almost as easy as changing your shirt these days—take advantage of it.

Hair Color

A shade close to your natural hair color will probably suit you best. A good idea is to avoid drabness; gray hair is not your enemy, drabness of the hair that has not yet turned gray is. Harsh colors that contrast too much with the natural skin color, whether white, red, blonde, or black, require more striking features and personality types than the softer, more natural warm shades. Natural gray hair can be strikingly beautiful, on men and women.

You Can Do It Yourself

If you hate going to the hairdresser, learn to do it yourself. You can have it cut so that it is easy to care for. Always, repeat always, keep your hair sparkling clean. Unwashed hair is terribly depressing to the spirit, and if you've been afraid that frequent shampoos would increase a baldness problem, don't worry; they won't.

Baldness

Millions of dollars are spent each year on baldness cures, but except for recently developed hair transplants, none have proved successful. Three channels are open to balding persons.

1. Get a wig or toupee. The cost is not unreasonable, and they work instantly, whether your goal is to compete on a more even basis with young people on the job, in romance—or just to make you feel good. See preceding paragraphs on color. Men do not need to worry as much as women about harshness in color and line, but avoid the totally unnatural.

2. Try a new hair style, or several hair styles. Go to a different barber or to one of the many men's hair stylists that are springing up in numbers all over the country.

3. Shave off all your hair and keep it shaved. This makes some men very pleasing to women, a sign of virility. There is nothing ordinary and timid in this step, and it may be better than wispy hair. You can always let it grow back.

Also for Men

Beards, sideburns, goatees, can revitalize your appearance at any age and are fun to wear. Experiment with these to complement your hair style. Find out what suits you and feels right to you, and remember that if you don't like it, you can always try something else.

Skin

When we think of youth we think of a skin that glows with health and that is supple, moist, and free of wrinkles. There are several factors that contribute to a healthy skin.

General health is important. See your doctor twice a year. *Exercise* flushes impurities from your skin by increasing blood circulation. *Good food* is necessary for renewing tissues. *Thorough and unrelenting attention to cleanliness* cannot be stressed too much. This is repeated so often because it is absolutely necessary; too many people of all ages still ignore this simple elementary necessity of a good-looking skin. Don't be one of them!

Skin shows age because oil and moisture is lost beginning at an early age, causing wrinkles to develop. Women suffer from drying skin more than men because of different hormones. Sunshine is our worst enemy—stay out of it or wear a covering make-up or cream that screens out burning rays. Sunshine makes the skin dry and leathery and intensifies wrinkling. It breaks down elastic fibers within the skin and can lead to discoloration and permanent damage, even skin cancer. If you must take sun baths or work outside, try to make it before ten in the morning or after three in the afternoon when the damaging rays of the sun are not so prevalent, but its tanning rays are still effective.

If you are not convinced that the sun ages your skin drastically, make this test. Compare your skin in areas that are normally covered by clothes with those areas that are not. The time to act is now, whatever your age, and remember that snow is a powerful reflector of the sun and that cloudy days can be deceiving. Also, that an umbrella at the beach is not enough because of the reflections of sand and water.

For general use for dry skin, a lanolin-enriched body lotion is indispensable and inexpensive. Use it on your arms and legs and any dry areas by wetting your hands with hot water, then pouring the lanolin lotion in your hands and rubbing it on the dry skin areas.

To improve skin tone and color, lie with your feet twenty inches or so higher than your head for fifteen or twenty minutes. This is a good pick-up when you're tired. Boards can be bought for this purpose, or you may use an ironing board propped up or lie on the bed or floor with your feet propped on the wall or a chair and a couple of pillows under your buttocks. The goal is to increase the flow of blood to your head for rejuvenating results.

Make-up

USE A MOISTURIZER AND LUBRICANT

Before applying make-up, use a moisturizer to lock in your own natural moisture during the day. Apply it only to clean skin and wait five minutes or more to put on make-up, otherwise the make-up will mix with the moisturizer and make the skin "dirty" again. A moisturizer does not take the place of a lubricant. Lubricants should be smoothed on your face and throat at night after cleaning your skin and let stay for fifteen minutes; then remove, otherwise your skin won't be able to breathe while you sleep. Because the skin around the eyes is particularly delicate and subject to wrinkles from drying, be sure to apply an eye cream, preferably one without a scent, as perfumes can cause puffiness in the tissue surrounging the eyes.

HEAVY CONCEALING MAKE-UP

Don't use it—it may work for the very young but not for

women whose skin has begun to dry (anyone over twenty). Avoid "dramatic" make-up as it is too harsh and will only make you look older. Heavy make-up fills in crevices and wrinkles, accentuating them rather than concealing them. To cover flaws, use a cover make-up very lightly on the flaws only and then blend it in to the surrounding areas. Better leave the throat free of make-up, as it can emphasize creping or sagging. Use a translucent powder instead of the caked kind, and use it sparingly.

EYE MAKE-UP

Eye make-up is especially effective, and the array of products offered can be staggering. Start with the basics—a tinted shadow, eyeliner, and eyebrow pencil. Softness is again the rule; always avoid harsh lines in make-up if you want to look young but particularly in eye make-up. You don't want to hide the "you" that your eyes express. Blend eye shadow so that it fades away at the edges of the eye area. Eyebrows are better with just light penciling; use short strokes, not a heavy drawn line, trying a gray pencil rather than dark brown or black. Experiment with the shape of the eyebrows. A gracefully curved arc is best for some people, while a shorter thicker brow suits others. Special magnifying glasses and mirrors are available for people who need them. False eyelashes can be terrific and make you feel glamorous when the occasion calls for it. Extra long thick lashes could be too harsh, defeating your grow-young purposes. You may prefer to use mascara and curl your own lashes. If you have a beauty salon that you like, the operator will help you select lashes and show you how to apply them.

Color for Your Face

On sallow-toned skin, warm tones are better than the blue-ish reds. Try coral shades. The skillful use of rouge and blushers helps tremendously. Try adding rouge to the forehead and chin as well as to the cheek and blend so that almost the whole face is brightened with color. Practice and experiment until you find the key to your own best face.

Face Lifting and Cosmetic Surgery

An alert and actively involved person is less likely to feel the need for surgery because he or she is less dependent on looks for a feeling of worthiness and youthful vitality. This is not to put down the value of plastic surgery, however. For many people a youthful look is a necessity of their job, and for those who can afford it, it certainly does make a difference. (Incidentally, a famous plastic surgeon once said that the three chief enemies of middle-aged women are too much sun, too much alcohol, and not enough sleep.)

In face lifting, most frequently the skin is cut and literally "lifted," taking up the slack in the cheeks and jowls and leaving it firm and less wrinkled. The surgeon tries to hide any scars in the hairline. Results vary, but the basic lift should last seven to ten years. There is also a "mini-lift" that works well for those who have sagging only in the cheek and jowl areas.

Eye surgery, called blepharoplasty, removes fat and excess skin from the upper or lower eyelids and is fairly common among models and people in the acting profession.

Nose shape can be changed by rhinoplasty and is the most popular cosmetic operation performed.

Whole faces can be rebuilt by surgery and transplants performed for those who were born deformed or who have suffered disfigurement in accidents.

Other forms of surgery performed for those who want to improve their overall looks include operations to increase—or decrease—the size of the bosom. Excess body fat is sometimes removed by surgery, and legs that differ in size due to polio can be helped, also.

Plastic surgery sometimes is more disfiguring than beautifying if performed by a careless or unskilled doctor. If you should decide to have it done, do go to someone highly recommended by your doctor or ask a medical school in your area to recommend someone for the particular type of work you want done. And be prepared to have a change in your personality as well as your looks.

Disfiguring Marks

Scars, moles and discolorations can be helped, so that there's no need to put up with them if they detract from your good looks. Some famous beauties and unforgetably attractive men have been made more appealing by their leaving their disfiguring marks as they were—or even amplifying them. The eye patch, beauty mark, an interesting scar, these, like wrinkles, can make an ordinary-looking face a striking one. Your doctor can advise you about whether moles and other marks can be removed surgically. Dermabrasion by a plastic surgeon or dermatologist works, and chemical peeling may also work, but this last can be more harmful than helpful if not done by a highly skilled professional.

Special cover make-up is also available.

Excessive Facial Hair

In times past, facial hair was considered beautiful and desirable on women. It can be removed by wax or depilatory creams and by electrolysis. Electrolysis should be done only by a professional. The number of visits will vary depending on how stubborn the case is. Wax and cream depilatories can be used at home, or hair can be removed this way in a salon. If at home, experiment first on a nonexposed area.

Teeth

Everyone likes, and can have, a big wide smile without fear of exposing unsightly mouth problems. There has been great progress in dental techniques in recent years, and if your dentist is not one that keeps up with new methods, find one that does. The sooner you start, the better—and the less expensive it will be. Your looks will benefit tremendously, as well as your confidence and your general health. Replacing and recapping bad teeth is commonplace. Dental care now can save more difficult cosmetic repair later since the lines, bones, and contours of your face are all closely related to the jaw line and what is inside your mouth. Ask your dentist specifically about gum-tissue problems; these can be the cause of more loss of teeth than cavities and other dental problems. You'll be a great deal happier and healthier person by attending to your teeth now.

Hearing

Why mention hearing in a chapter on appearance? Because if you have trouble hearing it shows in your face, especially the eyes. You are likely to appear distracted and to have a blank look on your face. The major reason for getting help, though, is not for the sake of appearance but so that you will be able to converse normally and to be alert to what's going on about you.

Your Voice

While voice also is not part of appearance, it does affect your total image. It conveys emotions, your joy in living, your involvement or boredom, your youthful spirit or premature age.

How can you make your voice youthful? Mainly by being conscious of the fact that it, too, plays a roll in your grow-young program.

Here's how to listen to yourself. Cup your hands in front of your ears, palms backward. Now talk. Another trick is to stand in the corner of a room, with your face about a foot away from the corner, and talk.

No matter how you sound now, what you're after is a pleasing voice. Put your hands on your chest, over the breast bone, talk and you should feel vibrations. Now pitch your voice lower, now higher, keeping your hand on your chest, attuned to the vibrations. A vibrant voice is one that vibrates—that's it. Through practice you can make this pleasant low-pitched vibrant voice your normal speaking voice.

Posture, again, is an important factor in the way you speak. Great singing and acting voices vibrate lower down in the chest and the abdomen. Deep breathing exercises are beneficial, as are exercises such as walking and swimming.

In addition to voice timber and vibrating qualities, voices have color. Some are monotonous, dry, dull, and boring to hear even if the words are interesting. Through awareness, you can add color to the way you speak, variety in inflection and tone, rhythm, staccato, softness, crispness, firmness, enunciation—all of these make your voice more interesting, and you a more interesting person. Avoid speaking with a harsh, shrill, piercing voice; you'll be rewarded in ways you never thought possible.

Eyeglasses

If you need to wear glasses and don't because you think they are aging, better consider this: Your looks will suffer more permanently from squinting and frowning, causing unerasable wrinkles, than from wearing glasses or contact lenses.

Glasses are not an "old age" item; they are worn by numerous teenagers and youths in their early twenties, whether they need them for vision or not. By all means don't hesitate to wear them if you need them. Even if you don't need them, they can lend glamor to your appearance, particularly in the tinted lenses and bold frames.

Prescription lenses can now be set in the stylish frames. Experiment to see what color and shape of frame suit you best. Consider a darker frame and also the new styles available in metal frames. Don't settle for the same old-fashioned glasses!

Contact lenses have become easier to wear, and your ophthalmologist will advise you whether you can wear them. Not everyone is successful, but a great many more people are successful now than when they were first introduced.

Clothes

Clothes are enjoyable; style, color, line, tailoring, can produce the equivalent of a work of art, or an extremely fine hand-crafted object. Fabrics are to be appreciated for their sensuous qualities. What is nicer to touch than a sweater hand-knit of natural wool, silk, satin, or English tweed! Browsing in the fabrics department in a store or in ready-to-wear can be as exciting as a visit to a museum. And you can wear almost any of them—with spirit!

One of the easiest ways to feel young and look young is

through your choice of clothing. Never have we been so free to wear almost anything—all it takes is a bit of flair, which can be learned. Clothes can exhilarate us or depress us, make us look young or look old. Should you go way out? Play it safe and use clothing as camouflage so that you blend into the background, unnoticed?

Before thinking about specific ways of dressing that denote youth, it's good to think about the psychology of dress. Clothes make a strong statement, no doubt about it. Think about yourself, the kind of life you lead. Think about some of the ideas and activities you are reading in this book. Now think about the kind of person you would like to be, what you would like most to do, how you want to look, your goals for five years from now, ten years from now. Elegant, active, cute, studious, involved, sedate? Country gentleman, man about town, career woman, garden-club president, TV host? Nan's mother, Helen's husband, John's parent? Use these as ways to define yourself, not as goals in themselves.

Color

This is the first thing people note. Highway signs are in color; children can distinguish color before shape. So, use color as a device—but don't forget that it is a device. When we think of age, we think of faded colors, gray, black, dark blue, or brown. There's nothing wrong with these colors if they are brightened with accessories or are used with exceptional flair. You'll feel brighter and look younger if you make good use of clear colors. They don't have to be glaring. Avoid harsh colors as the birthdays pass.

There are so many more colors these days than existed a few years ago, for men's as well as women's clothing. Try them all, and if you've always had the idea that you couldn't wear green or red, take a new look. The greens and reds aren't what they used to be and neither are the yellows, blues, and lavenders. The grays and browns have changed, too, so if you must stick to the basic colors for items such as suits or coats, explore the new shades of the colors usually thought of as drab. Go to stores and try then on—with an open mind. If you don't want to invest in an expensive coat or suit in the new color, experiment with a shirt or blouse or some other inexpensive item. What have you got to lose?

Fit

We associate age with baggy trousers, a dress that sags or just hangs from the shoulders shapelessly. Let's face it, they look droopy, dispirited, no matter what the age of the wearer. Just as unattractive is the appearance of the person who has put on weight and outgrown his clothes. Too tight clothing does not create a sexy look even if weight is no problem. Neither does clothing that is too loose. They won't fool anyone into thinking that you're the proper weight—whether under- or over-weight. If you want to grow young, see that your clothes fit well.

Length of Clothing

Try to keep fairly current with the styles, but avoid exageration. If you want to wear full length dresses or very short dresses at home when you feel whimsical, that's great—but you'll be labeled as trying too hard if you wear them on the street when everyone else wears more moderate lengths. What looks kicky on youngsters can look ridiculous after thirty.

Men should not wear trousers that droop around the ankles or waist. It takes an awful lot of charm, good looks, and spirit to overcome this one easily corrected fault. Put your charm to work in better ways and let your tailor take up the trousers.

Accessories

Shoes, hats, handbags, neckties, scarves, and belts, are great pick-ups for the spirit. Color (or bright white) can be wild in small doses, and accessories offer the perfect opportunity. Stylish boots, a bright silk scarf, handsome gloves, should not be overlooked as instant youth builders.

Rejuvenating Exercise—Without Boredom

For many people the term "exercise" has become a "turn-off" word, connoting boring, repetitious drills in which you mutter "one-two-three-four, reach-down-touch-the-floor" while you huff and puff in a mental vacuum and wonder how an intelligent adult ever got talked into this situation. Yet the term is a useful one, and instead of trying to concoct a fancy term to replace it, let's just smash the unfortunate image it conjures up and examine the reality, which is something different indeed.

What Exercise Is

Exercise is joy in motion, delight in the way your body responds to your command to move the way you want it to.

Exercise is dancing half the night with your best girl—or a strange man you met five minutes ago at a party.

Exercise is playing sandlot baseball with the neighborhood kids.

Exercise is clearing a space behind the house to plant a small garden.

Exercise is walking from antique shop to antique shop in search of a chair to replace the one that collapsed yesterday.

Exercise is water-skiing on a Minnesota lake. Exercise is playing Ping-Pong with your husband on the dining room table.

None of these activities conform to the one-two-three-four image of exercise, yet each is just as beneficial. And since they are fun, they are much more likely to be repeated often enough to bring the results you are after. One-two-three-four exercises work, too, but it takes more determination to keep at them. We want to structure liveliness and fun into our lives, not repetitious boredom, so we will leave instructions for those exercises to other sources.

The Results You Can Expect

Exercise invigorates the glandular system—and the glandular system manages the aging process.

Exercise causes the chest measurement to expand and the waistline to reduce—the reverse of the usual aging sympton of sunken chest and outthrust abdomen.

Exercise reduces tension and is therefore good for our mental health.

Exercise gives you self-confidence.

Exercise can help you loose weight.

Exercise can help you to redistribute weight—it converts fat to lean muscle.

Exercise can help prolong your life for a number of medical reasons, the most important of which is probably by reducing greatly your chance of heart disease. It helps the heart pump life-giving blood and nutrients through your body and flush away wastes. Muscles in action force the blood along, thereby giving your heart a needed helping hand. It increases the capacity of the heart to stand stress and helps keep the blood vessels free of obstruction, thereby reducing the chances of a stroke. It increases the capacity of the lungs and the ability of other vital organs to perform so that your body stays in balance and is able to resist infection, disease, and the wear and tear of everyday living.

Exercise helps you to move gracefully, bringing admiration from others.

Exercise increases your ability to react, helping you to avoid accidents.

Exercise produces better posture, subtracting years from your appearance.

Exercise is good for curing the blues.

Exercise is conquest over sloth and indifference.

Exercise increases your metabolism (the rate at which you consume your food intake), thereby helping you lose weight.

These are but a few of the good results you can expect; there are many, many more.

What If You Don't Exercise?

That's a fair question. Perhaps it is best answered by observing the people you see or know of who don't exercise. Excess weight, unhappiness, poor color, poor appetite, weak muscles, short breath, lack of joy in living—and premature age. Resulting bad posture affects your mental condition, the health of your kidneys, reproductive organs, lungs, and brain.

Also, consider this: About 50 percent of all heart attacks occur during sleep; only 2 percent while active.

Getting Started

When do you start?

Now, whatever your age.

When do you stop?

You don't, not when you are sixty or eighty. Motion is

life.

First examine the objections to getting started, and then shoot them down, one by one.

"Exercise is boring."

> You weren't bored running, jumping, swimming, or playing games as a child, and that was exercise. If routine exercises bore you, select from a wide range of others that will give you the results you need while also bringing adventure and new friends into your life.

"After working around the house (or on the job) all day, I'm too tired to exercise."

> Tired of what? Of housework? Of your job? If you suffer from the same fatigue of which millions complain, doctors say it is more likely brought on by boredom with the tasks or resentment at having to do the work than by muscular effort. Following your workday with a half hour of exhilarating and enjoyable exercise (volleyball?) will actually take away the fatigue and restore your energy.

"After all these years, I'm not in condition. Just don't have the stamina or the will power."

> You get into condition by starting gradually; you develop the will power by starting today. Make the one big effort to get started—and then capitalize on your investment day in and day out.

"I don't have the extra time."

> You don't need extra time. Just use part of your time each day differently. Twenty minutes a day stolen from the television set; twenty minutes a day walking instead of riding; fifteen minutes a day stretching instead of slouching. That's the start of a ritual that puts you on the road to growing young and changing your life.

"I'm not as young as I used to be. Have to slow down a bit."

> Who said so? Ask your doctor if exercise will hurt you. If

he gives you the green light, immediately get out of the "slow down" aging trap and start living. Deprive your body of the exercise it needs and it will retaliate by displaying all the signs of premature age.

When You First Start

Get an okay from your doctor. He will advise you whether you can undertake very strenuous exercises.

Don't rush in and play tennis your first time out. Start gradually, even with walking. Wait a few days after your first round to give your muscles time to recover.

Remember that exercise is not something you will do for eighteen days for results and then quit.

Exercise must be a part of your routine for all of your grow-young life.

You Can Do It Alone

If group activity is not feasible, make the plunge on your own—now. Resolve to get off the train or bus one station before your normal stop and walk the rest of the way home. Set your alarm half an hour earlier for tomorrow and spend fifteen minutes practicing your golf swing.

Once you have gone three days in a row carrying out your resolve, bask in your victory. You deserve to give yourself a pat on the back. You have proved that you can overcome sloth, laziness (which we all suffer from to a degree), and despair. "Is it really worth the effort?" the enemy of youth within keeps nagging. You have to let it know who's boss. You're on your way.

Walking Is Taking Steps to Change Your Life

Walking has become the pastime of aristocrats. Everybody rides—to work, to the shops, to the theater. Only a few privileged people walk.

You can observe these aristocrats in every city and village. At any age, they stand out from the crowd, men and women in their thirties, and seventies, striding gloriously along, head up, eyes sparkling, complexion clear. Every movement conveys an image of physical well-being. Whatever their job or economic status—secretary, factory worker, executive, grandmother, intellectual—they are clearly among life's winners, for they have rolled back the years and broken through to the experience of a rich and fulfilling existence.

There's no need to envy these aristocrats. You can join them when you take part in this most enjoyable and exilarating of all renewal exercises. You don't have to follow the paths of noted walking tours through Scotland and Wales or hike the length of the Appalachian Trail—although I can't think of a better way to spend a vacation. The privilege of walking can be indulged "within walking distance" of your home.

What is so great about walking as a renewal exercise? Walking is a human activity, one of the few we are still permitted to perform in public in this age of mechanization. When we walk, we perceive people and things with an immediacy and wholeness not available from the throughway or the sky. Walking stimulates our curiosity and restores a sense of proportion to our lives—while benefiting our body.

Walking is sheer visual pleasure. Indulge it with an acquaintance, and under the stimulus of sights and sounds you will find yourself rapidly turning into a first-rate conversationalist.

Walk alone, staying off the highways and exploring the byways—streets you may have passed through in a car or bus but never bothered to observe closely, woods and fields where nature delights your senses with a never-ending spectacle.

Walking builds self-confidence. Stride briskly along, head up, shoulders back, and you will find the above-the-crowd image you give to others reflected back to you in admiring glances.

Walking is enjoying your body in motion. It is getting out and doing something even when you don't feel up to it. It is striding over boredom and tedium and defeat into victory.

What Walking Does

Walking slims your body and firms your muscles, curbs sagging and flabbiness. Result: a more youthful and appealing body.

Walking tones up your heart and circulatory system, benefits your kidneys and stomach, your lungs and brain.

Walking increases your metabolism. You burn up calories at the rate of about five per minute when you walk at a speed of four miles per hour. While enjoying the pleasures of walking, you lose weight—without dieting! A thirty-minute walk consumes up to 150 calories.

Walking stimulates circulation, which helps you to attain and maintain a clear, youthful complexion.

Walking relieves tension, anger, frustration. Under the strain of on-the-job and family tensions or continuing mental activity, the blood vessels contract. Walking dilates these vessels.

Walking transforms your body into an alert and alive system for total living.

How to Walk

It is a sad commentary on our civilization that adults need to be taught to walk, Mostly, we push agitatedly through a crowd or move listlessly with our legs only, leaving the rest of the body uninvolved. How few of our steps are infused with the buoyancy and rhythmic swing of joyful walking.

Begin your new regimen with moderation. At a brisk pace, walk steadily for fifteen minutes each day. Don't stroll. To qualify as a grow-young exercise, walking should be vigorous, causing you to huff and puff a bit and your heart to race. (If you have a heart condition, check with your doctor before undertaking any exercise program.) This training of your heart muscles and respiratory system is one of the goals of walking.

Gradually increase the duration of your walks—from fifteen to twenty minutes and then to half an hour. As you break down the old sedentary habits, you will actively seek out occasions for longer and longer walks—both for the sheer pleasure of the activity and the grow-young credits you accumulate in this way.

If walking half an hour at a time isn't practical, break up your day into walk intervals. You will be pleasantly surprised at the refreshment you bring back from the ten-minute walks with which you intersperse your day.

Walk with head up and shoulders back. This will give you an unnaturally rigid appearance the first few times you attempt it. Don't worry. You are merely proving to your body that bad walking and posture habits can be conquered—that there are alternatives to walking in an aging slouch. After a week of this posture training, begin relaxing a bit. You will find that your old way of walking no longer satisfies you. You have moved into a new and grow-young pattern.

Walk with a purpose, to the shops, to explore a different scene, to visit a friend, to see what's happening on the other side of town, to see if the wild roses are in bloom. Build walking into your life.

Walk comfortably. Special walking togs aren't necessary, just comfortable shoes and easygoing clothes. Tight-fitting garments that interfere with circulation are no good at any time. They are completely out of place when you walk to reinvigorate your body.

On the other hand, don't underestimate the psychological power of a handsome walking stick to add a certain swagger to your gait—or of a colorful blouse and pair of slacks to put a spring in your step. Walk joyously into your new life—and carry whatever plumage makes you feel good. People will only admire your independent spirit.

What happens if you skip a day during the week? Nothing disastrous. Certainly there's no cause to build up guilt feelings and taint your entire renewal effort. Whenever you do feel tempted to slacken off, reread the preceding pages on the purpose and rewards of exercise. Once more get your goals in focus: a healthy, vigorous, and attractive body.

Look where you walk, perhaps you are mechanically following the same route every day and at the same hour and are thus getting a bit bored. Then vary the spectacle, explore new vistas, feast your senses on different people, woods, hills, streets, buildings. Make of each walk a voyage into the unknown from whence you return with a treasure-trove of new impressions. No wonder great walkers are often great talkers and entertaining writers. Within walking distance, they find the world for observation.

Jogging, Swimming, Bicycling

Jogging has its advocates. I am not one of them. A rather grim and joyless means to an end, it offers few interim rewards to the participant—or the spectator. It is difficult to fit into the normal day, and as a routine it breaks down under the demands of daily life. Jogging is a "special situation" exercise; walking you can indulge in at any time and anywhere, and it is safer and certainly as beneficial to your bodily system as jogging.

Dancing, swimming, bicycling, and other sports that offer fun in the doing will slim your figure, tone up your body, improve your complexion, and enhance your overall sense of well-being. Obviously, they are wonderful for grow-young activities.

Most of the blocks to enjoying renewal through sports are psychological rather than physical. That's because sports are associated with competitiveness. Unless you can win or perform better than the next person, you don't want to play. That's understandable. But the pools and beaches are crowded with inexpert "swimmers," and the amateurs far outnumber the golfing pros. Find out which sport appeals to you most—not just the physical activity but the social ambiance, also—and then plunge in with the other amateurs. Once you have broken the shyness barrier, lack of skill won't deter you from joining in—and improving.

But if a particular sport—or all sports—bore you, admit it. Not everyone is a sports buff. There are plenty of other enjoyable opportunities around for conditioning your body.

Go dancing. Buy a bicycle. But get moving somehow in a way that you enjoy.

We cannot grow young with grim determination. We have to expand our mind and body and spirit through exhilarating involvement and action.

Food for Pleasure and Vitality

Pleasures, as this book repeatedly emphasizes, are necessary for growing young. And for most of us food is certainly one of the major sources of pleasure. If it isn't, we are missing out on one of life's enduring delights.

When we look back on our childhood and teens, food is one of the things we remember best. It is rich with associations, and the taste of a favorite food can suddenly bring to our minds in a rush of almost total recall the emotions and events of times past.

Food not only nourishes our bodies for day-to-day living. It rebuilds tissue and helps us to grow young—at practically any age. "But it's too late for me, I'm too old for that," people sometimes protest. They are wrong, however, for diet therapy possesses tremendous restorative powers. Hair, eyes, and skin that have grown dull and lifeless can most certainly be rejuvenated. So why not start today to grow young the enjoyable way and change your eating habits to meet your needs?

The Pleasures of Eating

Before getting into the subject of nutrition and weight loss, let us examine some of the pleasurable grow-young aspects of food preparation and eating.

Our social life benefits immeasurably from good food. Throughout the centuries, kings, presidents, and diplomats have used food to encourage sociability, conviviality, and a sense of shared well-being.

Good food eaten in a pleasant atmosphere is relaxing. It breaks down barriers, banishes mistrust and fear, and sets the mood for acceptance, friendship, romance. One of the most sensuous of our daily activities, food should be relished and not just swallowed because we must hold body and soul together. To overlook the opportunities for pleasure and sociability offered by food that is well prepared and served is a sad waste of one of life's true gifts.

For men and women alike, food and its preparation can be an absorbing and rewarding interest. Some argue that all the world's great chefs have been men, and others say that all the great cooks have been women. Either way, food yields immense rewards in enjoyment and creativity.

Preparing food is a challenge to our intellect and skills. It is also a way of communicating with others. In nourishing others we give love, pleasure, reassurance—and sometimes life. It is true that today we can all go out and buy a meal. But seldom are these meals as good as those prepared by someone who wants to please us.

Indeed, the challenge of buying a good meal in a restaurant is greater than that of preparing it oneself. Not that we should pass up an occasional opportunity to eat out. A change of scene and routine is always beneficial.

The Pleasures of Cooking

Never have there been so many opportunities for learning to be a good cook or for bringing a revitalizing variety to our meals. In most places fresh fruits and vegetables are available the year round, and in great variety. Supermarkets abound with choices—and you can also grow your own.

There are thousands of cookbooks to choose from, and hundreds more are published each year. If there is a problem, it is one of selection. Ask acquaintances who are good cooks to make several recommendations and then browse through them in the bookstore before you buy. A good basic cookbook is *The Joy of Cooking* by Rombauer and Becker. Craig Claiborne, James Beard, and Julia Child have written very popular volumes. *The Fannie Farmer Boston Cooking School Cookbook* has also gained considerable fame. Your favorite home-service magazine may have several cookbooks in print. In addition, you may want to consult the paperbacks where you will find books on every cooking speciality imaginable.

Spend some time selecting a good cookbook. And start to read the recipes in the newspapers and magazines, clipping and filing those that appeal to you. If you have not already explored good food, expect to discover a world of good eating and many pleasurable hours ahead.

A Little Wine and Atmosphere

The pleasures of eating are enhanced by good wine—another challenge if you decide to become a connoisseur. But don't be thrown by the details of year and region that sometimes surrounds wine selection. You learn by tasting. So just take home a bottle without concerning yourself with vintage or rarity. If you enjoy it, go back for more. Keep experimenting until you find one that pleases you.

Music and candlelight, good company that you should try to vary almost as often as the menu—these, too, contribute to the pleasure of eating, as does the way you eat. This means treating food and alcohol with the respect they deserve, eating slowly, savoring every bite, pausing for converstion. If you are eating alone, try listening to records instead of watching the news on television. Browse lightly in a book instead of reading the newspaper. Between courses, read a poem several times, slowly, and allow its rhythms and images to mix with the pleasure of eating good food.

Sins Against the Pleasures of Eating

Make an effort to eat leisurely and without tension and you will benefit your disposition and digestion as well as enhance the enjoyment of your meal.

We often wonder why our bodies give us trouble, grow prematurely old, and cease to conform to the image we have in our mind. But consider some of the punishments many of us inflict on our bodies at mealtime:

> Eating while the television set assaults our eyes, ears, and nerves. That is like trying to appreciate a Mozart quartet in the midst of a traffic jam when all the horns are blowing at once.
>
> Use the occasion to try to close a big sales deal or make an impression on the boss. Wheeling and dealing, we push food into our mouths and swallow it with our nerves on edge. If you must make lunch or dinner the setting for business, try to settle the matter before actually eating—or hold it over until after. Avoid rich, spicy foods and keep alcohol intake to a minimum. Don't worry about appearing to be unable to "hold your liquor." Chances are your business associates will admire you for your courage in not drinking the way they do. If you feel you must explain, just say, "I save my drinking until after dinner." Try it. You will be surprised how easily it works.
>
> Use the occasion to settle family differences or recount the angers and frustrations of the day. Bickering at mealtime eventually causes you to have negative emotional associations regarding food and promotes unhealthy eating habits. Not only should you lay down the law and refuse to take part in this indigestion-producing talk, but you can take a positive approach and prevent it from arising. Be ready at meal time with interesting and entertaining things to talk about, amusing incidents observed during the day.
>
> Use food indiscriminately as solace for unhappiness, loneliness, frustration. Instead of relieving the situation, we aggravate it and to our other worries add obesity and poor health, thus starting a vicious cycle. (Food can give us an emotional boost, but when we build up a dependence on

food for this kind of support, we run into serious trouble. See the following sections on diet.)

Use food to bribe someone or curry favors or love, serving rich dishes that provide little real nourishment for those we care about.

Today, we have an abundance of good food that all of us can learn to prepare well. Budget foods cooked with imagination and care are better than expensive foods carelessly cooked and served. Wines and candles and music, too, are inexpensive. With all of this bounty on our hands, let us not abuse the occasion of eating but make it as pleasurable and relaxing as possible.

The Problem of Diet

Diet foods can be enjoyable but require extra thought. If your doctor has recommended a special diet, whether because of your physical condition or because you want to lose weight, be sure to ask him what "diet enliveners" you are allowed. Salt or fats may be prohibited, but there are many kinds of herbs he may encourage. Your doctor realizes that the more you enjoy your diet, the more likely you are to stick with it.

Explore herb cooking and spices and the dozens of flavors that can be purchased in small bottles: almond, vanilla, the fruit flavors, oriental seasonings, the regional specialties of foreign lands. Diet foods may be necessary, but it's not necessary that they be dull.

So much has been written about overweight that those of us who are underweight have cause to feel neglected. Since so little is published about underweight conditions, we may be misled into thinking that no nutritional problem exists. Actually, tipping the scales below the suggested weight for your body demands a re-examination of eating habits as much as does excess weight.

Fortunately, you can do something about an underweight condition if you start now. Write down everything you eat and drink each day for an entire week, skipping nothing. Then compare the food values you are getting with the nutritional information in this book.

Take your list of foods to your doctor. It will assist him in recommending a more healthful diet. Perhaps he will suggest ways to perk up your appetite if that is your problem. Exercise and fresh air will do much to give you a healthy, hungry feeling as mealtime approaches, as will mental activity, involvement, leading a full life.

Most of our food habits are deep-rooted, patterns that we began to establish as babies. They are as much a part of ourselves as the way we walk, talk, and look at life. While we cannot change the past, we can learn more healthful eating habits just as we can learn new words or to walk with a better posture.

Additives, Supplements, and Vitamins

Worrying about the food we eat is understandable. The newspapers and magazines carry news about additives, supplements,vitamins, health and organic foods, special diets in bewildering variety. Not even the experts agree, Some doctors say that if you eat properly, vitamin and mineral supplements are unnecessary. Others are firm believers in their usefulness. There is probably some truth in both points of view: some of us may need a vitamin "assist," some of us may not. Our food problems are as varied as are our life styles and personalities.

Also, it is very tempting to permanently adopt the attitude that, "Oh, I'm taking my vitamins, so it doesn't matter what I eat." This can be dangerous because not all of the nutrients vital to our health have been classified and made available in pill form. A lot has been learned by scientists, but they admit they have a long way to go. Don't depend on pills for your nutritional needs. It's too important.

On the other hand, it must be recognized that many of us do not get every nutrient we need, every day, from our food. It is for this reason that many doctors recommend vitamin supplements and possibly iron.

Controversy continues to rage about large-quantity supplements of vitamins C and E, some specialists highly recommending them and others vehemently decrying their use. Too much vitamin D has been reported to be harmful.

The best advice is to eat the foods that provide the basic needs and to consult your doctor about vitamins and minerals.

Your Basic Foods

Here are the basic foods that adults should eat every day, according to information supplied by the United States Department of Agriculture, Cooperative Extension, Cornell University:

BREAD AND CEREAL GROUP

Four or more servings daily. Count as 1 serving 1 slice of bread or one biscuit, 1 cup of ready-to-eat cereal, 1/2 to 3/4 cup of cooked cereal. Bread and cereal must be whole grain or enriched, otherwise they do not count. Baked products, sweet rolls, etc., which are purchased unenriched, do not count nutritionally.

When bread and cereals are eaten along with milk or cheese, the protein is just as useful to the body as the protein in meat.

This food group furnishes iron and B vitamins. Iron is important for building red blood cells, which are especially needed by women. B vitamins help to change food into energy in the body. They also help keep the nervous system healthy and appetite and digestion normal

Breads and cereals are not necessarily high in calories. If you want to cut calories, don't add sugar, jelly, butter, rich sauces, etc., to these foods

Some packaged foods may or may not be enriched when purchased. Check the label to be sure. These include rice, macaroni, noodles, spaghetti, hominy grits, cornmeal, biscuit mix, and crackers. White bread and rolls (except sweet bread and rolls) are required by law in some states to be enriched, as are dark breads, cereals you cook, dry cereals, all-purpose flour, and self-rising flour.

MILK GROUP

The equivalent of 2 cups daily. Whole milk, dry, skim, buttermilk, and evaporated milk, drunk or used in cooked foods. The following milk foods have approximately the same amount of calcium as 1 cup of milk:

- 1 ounce of hard cheese
- 1 1/2 cups of cottage cheese
- 1 1/2 cups of ice cream

Milk is expecially important for calcium. Also it contains needed protein, riboflavin. There is no iron or vitamin C in milk.

MEAT GROUP

Two or more servings each day. One serving is 2 or 3 ounces of cooked lean meat, poultry, or fish. Two eggs count as one serving of meat, as does 1 cup of cooked dry beans or peas or 4 tablespoons of peanut butter.

The meat group is important for protein, iron, and B vitamins.

VEGETABLE AND FRUIT GROUP

Count as 1 serving 1/2 cup, raw or cooked, or 1 apple, 1 potato, 1/2 grapefruit, etc. All our vitamin C comes from this group and most of our vitamin A.

It is important that we have variety in fruits and vegetables because of the wide range of the nutrients they supply. Food in this group varies more than in the milk, meat, and cereal groups. For example, some fruits and vegetables have a large amount of vitamin C or A, but others have very little. Since vitamin C is not stored in the body, you must select foods that supply this vitamin every day. However, since vitamin A is stored, you need eat vitamin A foods only every other day.

Vitamin C dissolves in water and is destroyed when exposed to air, so those vegetables on which you depend for vitamin C should be cooked quickly in a minimum of water. (Save the cooking water and use it for cooking other foods.) Fruit juices, when opened should be covered and stored at once to protect them from air. Iron is not destroyed by cooking, although some may dissolve in the cooking water, which may be used again.

Foods especially important for vitamin C include:

- Citrus fruits and juices
- Juices from other fruits with vitamin C added
- Strawberries
- Cabbage
- Potatoes, both white and sweet, preferably cooked in the skin
- Dark greens
- Tomatoes and tomato juice
- Cantaloupe

Foods especially important for Vitamin A (1/2 cup is 1 serving, no less than every other day) include:

- Dark green vegetables, especially green leaves such as spinach
- Collards
- Beet greens
- Broccoli
- Endive
- Orange-colored vegetables and fruits (carrots, sweet potatoes, winter squash, apricots, cantaloupe)

Fruits and vegetables important for other nutrients:

- Dark green vegetables, especially with dark green leaves (iron and one of the B vitamins, also as above for C and A)
- Green peas and green beans (small amounts of iron but important if eaten often or in large quantities)
- Potatoes, both white and sweet (good sources of iron and one of the B vitamins. White potatoes are on the C

list, and sweet potatoes are on both the C and A lists.)

Other common fruits and vegetables that provide extra nutrients, calories, and add to the enjoyment of eating, but which are not outstanding for any one nutrient:

Corn
Head lettuce
Beets
Celery
Apples
Bananas

There are many additional foods not included in the four preceding basic groups: butter, oils, bacon, mayonnaise, candies, jellies, alcohol. These foods furnish calories—and eating pleasure. However, you should satisfy your needs first from the basic four.

Lean meat from less expensive cuts have just as much food value as the more costly cuts. Those of us who do heavy work do not need extra meat, but we do need extra calories, which can come from inexpensive foods such as bread and milk.

It is important to remember that one food taken alone may not supply the needed nutrient. Another food may be needed to activate it or make its nutritive qualities accessible to our body. Without sufficient vitamin D, for example, calcium is not used well by the body. For this reason, many forms of milk have vitamin D added. Check the label. (Apparently this is one of the vitamins that one can take too much of, so don't take twice as much as your doctor recommends, thinking that if a little is good, more is better!)

It should be apparent that there are many combinations of foods that will supply our bodies with the nutrients needed to replace tissue and build energy for joyful and youthful living. In variety is pleasure. So don't get into—or remain in—a food rut. Explore, experiment, and make of mealtime time a pleasurable, exciting, and rejuvenating experience.

Don't Let Overweight Age You

Is it possible to have too much of a good thing?

Certainly for the human system it is.

In this country, good food is plentiful and comparatively inexpensive. So are the labor-saving devices that reduce the demand made on our energy. Combine eating well with working less and the result is a hazardous health situation in which we take in more fuel than we have occasion to use.

The reverse side of the blessings of affluence and technology is overweight. We eat as though we walked miles to work each day and built our skyscrapers and superhighways with sheer muscle power.

To grow young, we must make the righting of this imbalance one of our major priorities. Fortunately, conquering overweight doesn't have to be a dreary and weary chore. It can prove to be an interesting and exciting part of your overall grow-young program.

Almost all overweight individuals have "gone on a diet" at one time or another. And while I hope that you will read this chapter in order to understand more about the problems of overweight and what to do about them, do not take it as advice to immediately plunge into a diet. For if you follow the guidelines in this book, you may lose weight without dieting.

You will become more physically active, thereby using up more calories.

You will become more involved and interested and thus less inclined to eat because you are bored.

You will enjoy food more, taking time to prepare it carefully and serve it imaginatively, and you will eat when you are relaxed.

You will take more pride in the way you look. Automatically you will cut down a little—because you have learned what a big difference a little effort can make.

Your motivation will be different six weeks or two months from now. So if you have tried dieting before and it didn't produce all the expected results, don't get hung-up on your entire grow-young program by beginning again now. Wait until the other guidelines have led you to a more confident stage and then start a really successful dieting program.

Food and Energy

To conquer overweight, we must first understand the problem. Many experts say that overweight people are usually poorly informed about the basics of nutrition. Most of us realize that we accumulate extra fat when we eat more food than our body requires to maintain its energy supply.

This energy is measured in calories, just as inches or miles are terms for measuring distance. Our bodies cannot function without energy (i.e., calories) because energy is needed to accomplish physical activity and also for the basic process of everyday living—the beating of the heart, the breathing of the lungs, body cells repairing themselves, new tissue growth, the production of heat to keep body temperature normal.

The energy needed to maintain these ongoing bodily processes is called the basal metabolic rate, or BMR. The BMR is affected by the composition of the body, age, and other factors. It increases while we are growing and decreases gradually during adult life. Therefore, we require less food as adults than in the growing years. If we want to consume the same amount of calories as adults that we consumed as a teen-ager, then we must compensate for the "growth" calories by additional physical activity.

Getting Started

Before embarking on weight reduction, it is important to set realistic goals. Otherwise, you will soon abandon the program. This leads to destructive guilt feelings ("failed again") and can sabotage your other grow-young efforts. So the key word is—realism.

It's also important to realize that the diet that works so wondrously well for one person may not work for another. Our bodies differ, and research has not yet disproved the influence of heredity and hormonal imbalance on weight.

Obviously, it is unfair to assume that all overweight people eat too much.

Many people who lose weight discover they are soon adding pounds again. One reason is misinformation about calories. They mistakenly believe, for example, that whole wheat, rye, or diet bread contain significantly fewer calories than white bread, when the content is actually about the same. Meat is thought to be low in calories because the charts give calorie counts for very small portions. Meat, however, contains considerable fat that cannot be trimmed away. And weight for weight, fat contains twice as many calories as carbohydrates or protein.

Another reason for regaining lost weight is that new eating habits have not become established. We revert to the pattern that caused the problem originally. We would not expect to be able to change overnight the way we walk or talk, yet we want a change in eating habits immediately.

Again, the key word is realism. People do learn new languages, exchange new habits for old, and you can change your eating pattern to achieve your weight reduction goal, but it takes motivation. And it takes action, the kind you will find recommended in practically every chapter of this book.

Appetite Controls

Appetite-controlling mechanisms have not yet been clearly enough identified to be of much help in weight reduction at this time. But we can build our own controls, working out eating patterns that carry us toward the desired effect.

For some, a regimen of five small meals a day may remove the pressure to overeat at any one meal. Others find they can cut down at each of three meals daily. The important thing is to find the plan that works most comfortably for you.

The miracle diets may work for a short time—but they won't change your eating style. Special combinations of fat, protein, and carbohydrates have been devised that promise quick and sure success, but experiments under controlled conditions have indicated that they produce no more weight loss than any other food intake with the same number of calories.

Drastic diet alterations of any kind can prove destructive both to your body and emotions and should not be undertaken without close supervision.

Once established, special situations that encourage overeating become difficult to correct. Women frequently believe they require extra food during pregnancy to support the growth of the fetus, forgetting that their decreased activity more than offsets these calorie needs.

Menopause, also partly because of decreased activity, is a danger period. And the depression that some women experience at this time may send them on countless trips to the refrigerator. The answer to this midlife depression is not of course to eat more, which only compounds the problem, but to ask the doctor for aid in overcoming the despondency.

After Thirty-five

Most of us tend to put on weight after we reach thirty five. Our living habits become set, and we fail to notice the weight gain until we have added fifteen or twenty pounds, at which time we may think it too much of a bother to take them off. And while we wouldn't think of carrying around every day a ten- or twenty-pound bag of sawdust, we uncomplainingly shoulder our own unnecessary load until a threat to our health jars us out of our complacency.

Unless we make a deliberate and persistent attempt to increase our activities after thirty-five, we must decrease our food intake or suffer the consequences. For one thing, at this stage in life most of us have access to many more labor-saving devices than in our teens. For another, there occurs a gradual reduction in our basal metabolic rate, which alone accounts for some extra weight. And as we progress into the thirties and forties, our active body tissue is gradually replaced with fat—even if our weight remains constant. Only by regular use of our muscles can we mitigate the onset of flabby tissue that usually results.

Also, in our thirties and forties we may encounter various dental problems and either consciously or unconsciously select only those foods that are easy to chew. Thus bread, cake, and potatoes replace the healthful role of crisp salads, fruits, and vegetables in our diet. This "easy way out" is really the easy way into a difficult overweight situation. What we need here is not easy-to-chew foods but teeth or dentures that permit us to eat grow-young foods.

Diets: Common Sense, Miracle and Otherwise

Crash diets should never be undertaken without the advice of your doctor. It's advisable to check with him also on diets that are intended to produce special results in a short period of time. Each body system is different, and what is right for one may be wrong for another.

On your own, study the nutrition section in this book and consult the calorie chart in your cookbook. Also get a small calorie pocket guide to carry with you. You can obtain *Calories and Weight, the USDA Pocket Guide* by requesting it from the United States Government Printing Office, Washington, D.C. 20402. Enclose twenty-five cents. It contains handy illustrations showing the size of slices of meat loaf or roast beef, for example, which go to make up "x" number of calories.

There has been extensive scientific research on ways to help those of us who are overweight. Chewing food slowly has been found helpful, as has group eating therapy. The dieters in this kind of effort relate to each other their emotional reactions to the individual foods they are eating. Thus they aid each other to understand why they are such compulsive eaters and for what emotional deprivation they are using food as a substitute.

So-called "miracle" diets may help us to take off a few pounds quickly. This has the advantage of giving us confidence to go on with the rest of our grow-young program and to continue dieting on a more moderate level. As long as the "miracle" diet is nutritionally sound and your doctor discovers no health condition that rules it out, there is no reason not to use it. But employ it only as a prop until you can switch to a more sensible eating regimen.

Some reducing programs, such as the Weight Watchers, accompany a strictly prescribed diet with the psychological reinforcement of "weigh ins." This has proved to be successful for more people probably than any other group diet plan. It is nutritionally sound, widely available, and inexpensive.

Calorie Facts

The following information on calories has been excerpted from *Calorie Sense and Nonsense*, published by Cornell University and the United States Department of Agriculture, Ithaca, N.Y.

ESTIMATING CALORIE NEEDS FOR ADULTS

Adults can make a rough estimate of daily calorie needs by multiplying their *desirable* body weight by:

16 calories if sedentary
20 calories if active
24 calories if very active (female)
29 calories if very active (male)

ABOUT CALORIES

1. All food calories are alike. Since calories are simply a unit of measure, calories supplied by cake are the same as those supplied by lettuce. Cake just furnishes many more of them in a usual serving.

2. All foods furnish some calories. Any food that

contains protein, fat, or cabohydrate furnishes calories when oxidized (burned) in the body.

Potential Energy Value	
carbohydrate (sugar or starch, for example)	115 calories per ounce
fat	255 calories per ounce

Foods with a high percentage of water (i.e., celery, lettuce, and spinach) have so little calorie-producing potential that they are usually disregarded as sources of food energy.

3. Treatment of food changes its calorie value only if the protein, carbohydrate, or fat content is changed. Thus toasting a slice of bread does not change its caloric value.

Calories and Action

Small activities add up. A typist can gain six pounds a year just by changing from a standard to an electric typewriter. Assuming a 15-calorie savings per hour, she accumulates:

90 extra calories per six hour day (450 per week)
22,500 extra calories per working year (450 × 50)
six additional pounds a year (22,500 divided by 3,500) (one pound body fat represents 3,500 stored calories)

With this information in mind, you can visualize how cutting down by just 90 calories a day (1 1/2 slices of bread) would reduce your calorie intake sufficiently to lose up to six pounds in a year. If you cut just one tablespoon of butter (100 calories), your loss would be greater.

Suppose you don't make even the minor cuts mentioned in the preceding paragraph? Then, depending on your present weight, you may add six pounds a year—and in three years that means eighteen pounds.

Just to maintain your status quo some control of eating habits is necessary. And if you combine a regular increase in activity with a regular cutback in eating, you will move way ahead in your grow-young program. You will look younger, feel younger, and think younger. Surely that is worth some effort?

More Tips on Weight Control

Bathroom scales are inexpensive. Buy one and use it once a week—not every day. It takes a week to register progress.

Curb unconscious eating. Gradually train yourself to be aware of every mouthful of food so that you do not automatically finish leftovers or snack as a ritual accompaniment to reading or watching television.

Suspect your motives. You may be entering a restaurant to eat when what you really desire is distraction, a chance to be with people, or a change of scene to break a despondent mood. You can find all of these things more easily at a movie, concert, park, or ride on a bus—and you won't put on weight.

Learn to anticipate your weak moments—the time you usually succumb to the temptation of a cookie. Get into the habit of eating some crisp celery, green pepper or a cup of steaming or iced boullion before that moment arrives. Try not to let yourself get overhungry; if you do you are bound to stuff yourself.

Find an alternative to boredom. Chances are you won't even think about eating when busily engaged in some activity that really absorbs you. This book lists several suggestions for activities and interests that can divert you from overeating because you have nothing to interest you.

Don't skip breakfast. A hearty, healthy breakfast reduces the chance of your eating a high calorie lunch and indulging in between-meal snacks. (If you're not hungry at breakfast, it may be because you consumed a few hundred calories worth of food before retiring the night before.)

Think about the texture of both new and familiar foods. Chew slowly and see if there are not nuances of flavor that previously escaped you. Experience the flavor and texture of a crusty piece of bread, of a potato with only coarse salt and pepper added. This extra awareness of food and your appreciation of basic flavors that had been disguised by rich sauces will more than compensate for smaller portions. And don't expect your new food selections and preparation techniques to duplicate the old. Green beans without the usual rich dressing is a new dish, not just the old served "without dressing."

Prepare food, vegetables especially, by cooking in as little water as possible until just tender.

Start with a one-day-at-a-time resolution. Tell yourself, "I can manage for just one day"—and you will. Then repeat the next day—and the next. After several of these one-day-at-a-time successes, you will have gained an impressive fund of confidence in your ability to change your eating habits.

When dieting, compensate yourself by indulging in some pleasure. Buy a new record, spend a weekend at your favorite place, add a new item to your collection.

Anticipate occasional moments of weakness and prepare for them by stocking the refrigerator with tasty low-calorie snacks. If all you have on hand is high-calorie food, that is what you will eat whenever you "have to have something." Stock lean meat, chicken without fat, fish, shrimp, boiled eggs, hard cheese, crunchy vegetables. Have snacks available that are already trimmed of fat and cooked ready at a moment's notice. Always include these foods in your shopping list. Repeat, always.

Make it a habit to plan your diet menu ahead. If you are undecided about food, the temptation to fall back on something familiar (and rich!) may prove overwhelming. Be prepared.

Learn to eat fruits raw. Fruits are not low in calories, but the uncooked are lower than sweetened cooked fruits. Include some in your diet every day.

Maintain your energy with a diet that is nutritious as well as low in calories. If you let your energy drop, you will convince yourself of the need for "quick energy"–meaning sweets.

Activity and exercise use up calories, make you feel more energetic, so that you will be more active all around. And that will use up more calories. Make this cycle work for you.

Since you are buying less rich expensive foods, you can afford to treat yourself to better quality fruits and vegetables, along with seasoning to add greater variety to your meals.

Remember it's the sensible diet that has the best chance of success, not the two-week wonder.

Make bland but nutritious and low-calorie foods tasty. For example: cottage cheese served with shrimp or clams and a sharp dressing–or with fruits sharpened with lemon or lime juice.

Investigate recipes for cold vegetable soups made raw with the help of a blender or food chopper.

Become a whizz at "budgeting" your calories. It can be as engrossing and rewarding as budgeting your money.

Accept another "budgeting" challenge. Equate your food intake with the energy you consume. For instance, walking daily one and three-quarters to two miles at a brisk pace consumes 156 calories. Swimming for thirty minutes with average skill uses up 336 calories.

Try to get rid of tension before meals. You will be less likely to gulp your food and overeaat. Divert your mind and quiet your emotions with one of the "Easy Starters" listed in this book. Make relaxing before meals a habit. See "A Time for Quiet."

Eating to roll back the years can be fun, once you realize that the nutritious foods your body requires to keep going and repair damages along the way are varied and tasteful enough to satisfy the most exacting gourmet. In a balanced diet, you can include the best of everything. Indeed, once you begin exploring the exciting possibilities of low-calorie nutritious foods, you will be likely to expand rather than limit your eating experiences. In food as elsewhere, the good things in life are to be enjoyed–even when dieting.

A Healthy Body for Growing Young

While our parents may have been locked into a life style that, for example, encouraged obesity, arteriosclerosis, and coronary prone behavior, today we have the options for a more healthful and youthful pattern of living clearly spelled out for us. Let us take advantage of the grow-young opportunities that science affords.

Because we may expect to live longer than previous generations in history, it is more important than ever to achieve and maintain good health. There is no point in living longer if our bodies are not up to enjoying those extra years.

A healthy body includes first of all attention to basic hygiene, regular medical checkups, moderation in eating and drinking, plenty of exercise, as much rest as our system requires, and cultivation of a cheerful disposition. Often the need to concern ourselves with these basic considerations gets buried beneath the headline-producing words such as heart disease, cancer, paralysis. This should not obscure their importance. Study your health habits to see if you are neglecting any one of them. If so, take corrective action now. Our bodies are such wonderful machines that it is very easy to overlook their basic needs–until they find it necessary to cry for help.

Most of us, whatever our present age, frequently bemoan the fact that we didn't do better by ourselves when we were sixteen or twenty-two or twenty-eight. Or that our parents didn't train us to have good posture or better eating habits or have our dental problems solved when we were still attending school. But that does not mean we can't do something about the situation now. As adults, we know what needs to be done, we know that the responsibility for doing it is ours alone, and we know that the means are available to help us.

Remember the best reason for starting now is that we will need our body machine for increasingly longer years, full of opportunities for actions blocked to our parents and grandparents.

The Wonders of Medical Research

Each day, researchers the world over add to an already impressive store of medical knowledge, converting one-time "killer" diseases into minor inconveniences, discovering vaccines, medicines, and surgical techniques and treatments for the remedy of practically every condition.

Almost as remarkable as the advances in fighting disease is the progress in preventive medicine, which means that medical science can now help us to maintain so healthy a physical condition that disease cannot easily obtain a foothold.

Billions of dollars are being spent throughout the world on research, research that is shared among nations, so that the people of France, for instance, can benefit from work done in Japan and Americans from work done in Sweden. Hundreds and thousands of workers are engaged in the study and application of ways to make humankind lead healthier and longer lives. We are even preserving and examining the medical lore of primitive cultures, for many of their herbs and curative practices are proving to be scientifically sound and not just "witchcraft."

Exciting discoveries are being made in the field of mental and emotional health, discoveries that often seem to reject the old idea that "it's all in your mind." Chemical substances, diet therapy, drugs, and a vast array of techniques are constantly being made available to the practicing physician for the purpose of helping all of us live better and longer lives.

Use the Advantages You Have

We can't afford not to take advantage of all these grow-young discoveries. Yet many of us live as though they did not exist or wait until damage to our bodies has reached a point at which cure becomes costly and difficult. We drag our feet because of fear, fear that something may be incurably wrong, fear that medical science cannot really help us, fear that the cost of the remedy will be too great. Instead of spending our days in living, we waste them in fear. We are afraid to play games, go dancing, or travel because we do not know whether or not our "condition" is up to it. So we deny our bodies the benefits of exercise, of exhilarating involvement, and build up situations of real stress that actually do cause illness–simply because we have imprisoned ourselves in a cage of worry.

The odds are that a physical examination will reveal nothing seriously wrong. If you do have a condition that needs correcting, modern medical science has perfected marvelous tools for remedying it. When illness forces you to visit a doctor, the cost and inconvenience can be high. When you go for regular checkups, you avoid the necessity for "crisis medicine" and benefit from common-sense maintenance programs. Don't put off going for a checkup any longer. Make an appointment today. It can be vital to your entire grow-young effort.

Where Your Doctor Can Help Your Grow-Young Program

In addition to diagnosis and treatment of illness, your doctor can advise you in important grow-young maintenance areas:

Prescribing a specific diet, whether you want to lose or gain weight, or for other physical conditions that make dieting advisable.

Determine your fitness level for an exercise program. Too often our enthusiasm is captured by a fad, and we plunge right in without learning if we are helping or hurting ourselves.

Help us to break out of a cycle of tension, driving ambition, insufficient rest, a coronary-prone life style. Your doctor can issue early warning signals against habits that may be making you prematurely old.

Help us to overcome the pressure of our neighbors and the solicitations of the media to consume more—more food, more drink, more tobacco, more mileage, more everything.

Reassure us that we are on the right track and that all is well so that we can participate fully in the life around us.

Help with emotional problems such as depression and anxiety.

Going Beyond Your Doctor

There are a number of large medical centers throughout the country where one can undergo a series of medical tests and examinations under the supervision of specialists. Medical schools and teaching hospitals frequently offer this service. Write for information to the one nearest you.

These health centers are prepared to determine any treatment you may need, as they are equipped with the most advanced technology for testing and evaluation. They can detect the hidden signs of an illness at an early stage so that treatment has a better chance of complete success. Because many specialists and much equipment are centered in one place, overall examinations are less time-consumng than visits to separate specialized facilities. Often they recommend that the actual treatment be carried out in facilities close to your area or by your own doctor. The tests may require more than one day, and the cost is usually more than that of a normal examination. But it is worth the time and money.

Don't waste your energy worrying about whether you are getting all the medical attention you need or whether your general doctor is overlooking some rare disease. Chances are he isn't, but if you want the additional reassurance, the means are now available for getting it.

Schedules

A healthy body needs continuous upkeep. But most repetitive tasks involved in bodily maintenance can get boring. That's why it is so important to build it into our daily routine.

Set a daily schedule of basic hygiene. Total cleanliness, rigorous attention to teeth, hair, nails, feet. Weigh in to monitor your food intake. Complete these tasks in a fixed order until they become second nature. That way you can perform them without a second thought–and without skipping any one, ever. Read the chapter on "Automating Upkeep."

Your Health Image

The way you see yourself affects your health. Those of us without grow-young goals who conceive of ourselves as life's victims have no interests and little to look forward to, lack the motivation necessary to build good health habits or even to remedy illnesses. Subsisting on "make do" foods, slouching instead of walking briskly, we systematically abuse our body until only major repair can set us right. This is sheer self-destruction, the death wish running rampant.

If you have even the slightest tendency to victimize yourself in this fashion, start to build a positive and healthful image of yourself today. Whatever your problem—overweight, poor vision, bad posture, drab complexion—this healthful image will serve as a launching pad for beneficial change.

Another big help for healthful change can come from putting more fun in your life. Enjoyment of life is not just a privilege, it is an obligation if we are not to waste the years that have been given to us. When we don't receive rewards from living, we start to lose interest and become resigned to what we mistakenly believe is "our fate."

It is difficult for our body to function well without the quickening of the spirit, without making demands on it, and without pushing it a bit in the business of life. Without these challenges, it atrophies. Love, joy in seeing a beautiful face or a flower, satisfaction derived from completing a job successfully—these and hundreds of ways in which we can reward ourselves are necessary for the healthy body we need to grow young.

Automate Your Upkeep

One of the telltale signs of premature age is personal neglect—not bothering with the admittedly tiresome details of everyday grooming and hygiene, skipping the household chores because "what's the use, no one will notice," disregarding the letter or telephone call.

Particularly when we lack strong motivation, have no one whom we want to impress, the rituals of everyday maintenance, physical, mental, and social, seem to loom as major challenges. We have to summon so much energy to perform these monotonous, unchallenging tasks that we wonder, "Is it really worth it?"

Emphatically it is. Begin to get careless about personal hygiene and watch your stock go down, not only with others but also with yourself. (Those old jokes about bad breath and body odor were firmly rooted in reality.) Forget about sewing that button on your jacket or finishing the hem on your skirt and the message you telegraph to the world is one of life falling into disrepair.

Of course you may have legitimate excuses for avoiding upkeep chores. And the next time you will have no difficulty in discovering more reasons for postponing them. Eventually, some of them drop out of your life completely. And so it goes until you reach the point where an effort to regain the respect of yourself and of others grows truly monumental.

As destructive to your grow-young program as neglecting grooming and personal hygiene is allowing your mind and attitudes to accumulate dust and grime through lack of attention. Here again you are confronted with the problem of those bothersomee and repetitive details of upkeep.

If only there were some way to whiz through those dull and boring chores in short order!

Well, there is.

Maintenance: The Modern, Easy Way

The secret lies in automating your upkeep.

In business and industry, many of the tiresome and repetitive tasks formerly performed manually have now been taken over by the computer. Machines are "programmed" to carry out whatever instructions are given to them.

You achieve a similar degree of time- and energy-saving automation when you "program" yourself to automatically follow a certain diet or corrective health routine, to take two examples. Instead of reaching for the caloric dessert, you automatically reach for a crisp apple. While you go through the motions (and quite effectively complete) some necessary but uninspiring task, your mind is released for more enjoyable activity—planning an interesting dinner, working out a problem connected with your work, trying out the foreign language you are learning.

Preparing a program is really very easy. For example, set aside a specific time on the most convenient evening each week for maintenance work on your clothes. Make a special effort to adhere to this schedule for three weeks. Soon you will no longer be worrying about finding time for this task or resent the hour you give to it. Indeed, it will have become as automatic as eating and sleeping.

As long as you continue to make special projects out of repetitive tasks, they will inevitably fatigue you. It's not just the work itself that gets you down, it's the dread of anticipation—and make no mistake about it, dread is aging.

Stop Brooding: You Have Better Things to Do.

Release yourself from dread by automating whatever unpleasant tasks face you. Instead of brooding on a critical telephone call or work project that you fear or dislike, determine to get it over with.

Tell yourself "My time is too important to waste in this way. So here goes!" Then plunge right in. The first time you win this victory, the tensions that have been building up within will relax. And this relaxation will show in the way you look, walk, feel.

But don't stop there. Automate your victorious procedure. Having done it once, there's no doubt you can do it again. The next time a similar situation arises, just plug in your "program" and confidently proceed.

All of us need to take some special actions to maintain our youthful image and vitality. With some it is exercise or diet, with others it is breaking out of our isolation and getting involved. The more effort we make to turn these exceptional actions into automated programs, the easier they become and the faster we reap results.

If you have to think about walking briskly and breathing deeply with each step you take, you will soon get bored. But set out at a brisk pace and breathe deeply because you have programmed yourself to this routine and the biggest part of your battle is won.

Automation and Crisis

All of us, sometime after thirty, engage in an existential confrontation with ourselves. The certainties that guided our lives up to now appear shaky indeed. Impenetrable mists shroud the roads that only yesterday extended so clearly and surely into the future. So many of the things we deemed important now seem trivial and scarcely worth the effort of preserving. The temptation to "let go," to abandon the tried and true regimen of good diet, good health practices, and good grooming appear overwhelming.

This again is where automation pays off. For one thing, these maintenance programs can function on their own, as it were, without intervention on your part. Even if your will power reaches a low point, your program keeps you performing the necessary actions to carry you through the difficult time.

Again, the self-discipline enforced by automation keeps you from crumbling under the impact of crisis in your life. A look in the mirror assures you that your body is in good shape, and you walk down the street with the same buoyancy as before. Gradually, sustained by these continuing programs, the wisdom of your body reasserts itself and once more places in perspective the psychological doubts and fears associated with crisis.

Body tone translates into psychological elan. On the sheer strength of your physical well-being, your self-imposed discipline, you deal with apprehensions and uncertainties as normal occurrences of all our lives and shrink them to manageable size.

Automating Good Maintenance

How do you begin to build good maintenace programs?

First, decide which programs will benefit you. The following are practically universal in their applicability:

Health care—including visits to the doctor
Diet
Exercise
Personal cleanliness, grooming
Care of clothes

Each of the above may be programmed for specific hours and days of the week. Once you have decided on a schedule and find that it works, stick with it. At first you may experience minor inconveniences, simply because you are not accustomed to routine. But after you have repeated it several times, it will become automated.

Look at it this way. The first week, the "cost" of automating is moderately high. The second week it drops signifcantly. By the fourth week, it's all "profit." Actions that at one time drained your energy, bored and annoyed you, now glide past rapidly and easily.

When an occasion arises that demands that you break into your automated routine, simply rewrite the program slightly. Move the visit to the hairdresser around from afternoon to early morning. Rise an hour earlier to inventory your clothes situation or use your lunch period to complete the exercises you usually perform in the evening. But don't allow more than forty-eight hours to elapse before completing the scheduled task.

Expand Your Programs

Here are some other programs to help you grow young :

> Each day, automatically give something of yourself to others: a word of encouragement, a smile, a flower from your garden. Recommend a film or a book you have enjoyed. Offer to help, express an interest in another's problem or life.
>
> Automatically do something new each day. (See the chapters on "Easy Starters.")
>
> Make the search for adventure a regular part of your existence.
>
> Every day, spend some time getting rid of destructive habits, negative attitudes.
>
> Each day, examine the good things that happened: the moment of pleasure you gave to another, the success you enjoyed in sticking to your diet regimen, the improvement in your posture, how good you looked in that new dress or jacket, the progress you have made in developing your

interests.

Learn something each day—add a new word to your vocabulary, explore a different street or a new shop, chat for a moment with the new employee in your office or at the supermarket.

Routinely, reward yourself—don't just wear that new pair of slacks, appreciate yourself with an admiring glance in the mirror; don't just bathe, luxuriate in a scented bath with a cup of tea or glass of wine. Buy that new book or magazine that excited your curiosity; drop in on that foreign film on the way home.

Involve your home in your life. Make it the place where people gather, where solitude offers positive enjoyment, where you bring the tangled strands of daily life together.

But, you will object, what have these actions got to do with automation? Most of them seem like extraordinary steps, not readily programmed into our lives. And that is true. However, what you do automate is the daily procedure, the routine action of each day seeking out an occasion for a kind gesture, a moment of adventure, a broadening of interests. So do we program ourselves to make each day more exciting and rewarding, to open our minds and our hearts to the opportunities for growth and renewal everywhere around us.

Conquering Loneliness

At one time or another, all of us experience the sense of being unneeded, unwanted, confined to an unwilling solitude that we call loneliness.

Sometimes the experience is transitory, occurring during those intervals when we are "at loose ends," with no project to occupy our minds and hands and with no goal to strive for. This we can manage.

But there is another kind of loneliness that descends on us like a black cloud and, remaining, gradually turns us into grim and bitter individuals, old before our time. Persistent and corrosive, this all-enveloping loneliness can afflict us whether we live alone or not—and at any age. There is no person more lonely than the one who sits across the room from another with whom all communication has broken down. This is more acute when the couple's entire life has been almost entirely centered on work and child-rearing and now suddenly there are no goals or interests to share. At this time, also, they begin to feel useless and as surplus because for twenty or thirty years they have literally been necessary for the survival of their children, and the let-down when their children become independent can be shattering.

What is so insidious about loneliness is the way it feeds upon itself. Since no one cares if we keep up with the times, maintain a trim, healthy body, develop new interests, why bother? Increasingly we armor oursleves with a defiant caution, proclaiming our invulnerability, concealing our deepest feelings lest we give an advantage to others. Unneeded ourselves, we make, "Who needs you?" our desperate rallying cry, thereby turning off those who could most help us. Wrapped up in our own misery, we fail to recognize that others are suffering from a similar ailment and that the other is trying just as desperately to hide behind a barrier of concealed feelings.

I Need You—You Need Me

Of course "we" all need "you" just as "you" need "us," but the language for expressing this need has been so heaped over with social custom, fears, and inhibitions that we tend to forget its very existence. Now is the time to retrieve it.

"I need you—you need me." These are the magic words that conquer loneliness by once more committing us to the flux of human existence, the daily give and take of human association.

Few of us can break a lifetime habit of reticence and emotional caution by saying outright, "I need you," or, "You need me." But we can roll these words around on our tongue, as it were, until they lose some of their formidableness—and in doing so we will find that once this is absorbed into our consciousness, we feel less lonely, more a part of humankind.

Mostly we are held back by a fear of rejection. An imagined rebuff freezes the words on our tongue. But suppose we start by using these words in a situation in which they are assured of a warm reception?

All of us, at every age, possess some human qualities, skills, and aptitudes that are desperately needed by others. The skill may be as simple as reading the paper aloud or just conversing with another for one or two hours a week. It may be as intricate as teaching another how to run a small business.

In every community there exist organizations, hospitals, groups, or individuals devoted to helping others who need more of your time and dedication than you can possibly give. It takes but a telephone inquiry to your local newspaper, church, or political organization to discover how to offer your services. And when you do volunteer, you say, in effect, "You need me," and the response is sure to be, "Yes, we need you."

"But I want personal friendship or love, not organized service!" Of course you do, but group service is the quickest and least painful way to cross the bridge between confused rejection and loneliness and warm personal relationships.

Whatever road it takes, helping others leads to connection, communication, person-to-person warmth, mutuality of regard, all of which are the opposite of loneliness. It is the summing up of the acknowledgment that has informed some of the world's greatest works of literature: "We are all in this together."

Once you realize that others need you, it becomes easier to admit that you need others. There are many ways of expressing this need—a request for help in some problem, asking another to join your "helping others" group, an invitation to your home or to lunch in a restaurant, offered simply because you would enjoy the company of the other. Better than words, actions like these convey the sentiment that the other is somehow important to you. And who does not like to feel needed?

Involvement: the Enemy of Loneliness

Both the man or woman whose partner is too wrapped up in business or other pursuits to notice the existence of the other, and the person who lives alone, have the same options for conquering loneliness: get busy, get moving, get involved.

Sometimes we feel that the cloud of loneliness engulfing us is so huge that any attempt to dispel it with such a mundane activity as gardening, adult education, or community affairs is just plain ridiculous. We are *profoundly* lonely—and here is someone suggesting a cure that we might attempt any day of the week. Certainly more drastic measures are required to bring about any significant change in our condition!

What we fail to realize, however, is that these first small steps mark the most significant progress we will ever make in breaking free of our cloud. Like the tiniest breath of air on a still and humid day, they herald the storm that will finally clear the atmosphere and open up the vistas of change and opportunity lying all about us.

In giving of our time and skills to others, in overcoming our shyness and feigned indifference and joining the local ecology club, in volunteering to ring doorbells for a political candidate, we rejoin the network of human relationships that constitute the fabric of civilization. Our involvement will bring occasional frustrations, impatience with our fellows, momentary resentment at unpleasant chores. But there will be little room in our lives for loneliness.

Positive Actions

The more purpose and direction we give to these first steps, the better our chance of rapid success. That's why it is best to search out positive situations, gatherings that have a function other than just bringing people together.

To continue with our examples (see "Grow-Young Action Projects" for many others), at the adult-education class, the political meeting, at the bike-riding meet, all of those present are infused with a common interest. Their opinions will vary, but they have agreed on a framework of discussion or activity.

Thus, in gatherings of this kind the problem of what to talk about with strangers never arises. You are "all in the same boat," and whatever you say about the subject at hand will be relevant. Nor do you have to be particularly knowledgeable to gain a warm welcome. That you share the interests of the group is sufficient, and remember that everyone there feels the need of the group, just as you do. There's a good chance that you will meet these same people again and again and in the same natural circumstances, encouraging deeper acquaintance. Finally, when even one or two people become enthusiastic about a subject of common interest, shyness barriers have a way of dissolving among the entire group.

(A word of caution. If you are hoping for romantic interest, seek a group of both men and women, with a majority of the opposite sex. On the other hand, don't enroll in a night class, for instance, that would be boring to you—you'll come off as totally unappealing. Enthusiasm and real interest must be the rule. Better to be in a group of your own sex that you're keenly interested in; a fellow member will admire your vitality and invite you to meet his sister, or brother.)

From being a spectator, you will move on to participation. When you hear a request for volunteers, raise your hand. Not every task may be completely to your liking, but you will have joined the team, and that is the important step. You have entered into the "I need you—You need me" network. One interest sparks another, and soon you will have to pick and choose from among the many opportunities and demands for your talents.

Keeping Up with Life

Alone, unappreciated, we can find hundreds of excuses for "letting go," not bothering about our appearance, allowing our mental muscles to grow flabby through disuse. What's the point of trying to look good or develop new interests when no one cares?

"Keeping up with life," however, acts as one of the most effective weapons against loneliness. Mentally and physically, it keeps our muscle tone at fine pitch. It gives us the resolve and the stamina to maintain a healthy body even if, for the moment, the only appreciative glance it gets is the one we give it ourselves in the mirror. It holds us to a daily regimen of reading the newspapers and magazines and watching the television programs about foreign affairs and fashions.

When we keep up with life, we maintain in good standing our membership in the social network. At any time, we are "ready to go"—ready to join in a discussion about politics, ready to put in an appearance at a social event, ready to enter whatever new "grow-young" activity appeals to us. Since we can discover few reasons to stay at home and feel sorry for ourselves, we meet opportunity with action.

Another bonus: Our blood, circulation, body tone, and color respond by keeping up, also!

Living Alone

Living alone need not spell loneliness. With just a little effort, we can make our home, whether a country estate or just one room, the hub of an exciting universe around which revolve people, events, ideas.

To live alone is to enjoy a unique sense of freedom. How else can you set your own schedule, walk around with no clothes on when the mood strikes you, indulge your most outrageous decorative fancy, invite a friend in at a moment's notice, work away at your hobby all night long if you want to?

Alone, we can put ourselves to sleep with a Mozart symphony, spend hours pampering ourselves in a scented bath, overnight transform a brown study into a multihued world of exotic patterns and designs.

"A room of one's own" has been the age-old dream of writers, artists, and composers who sought just a few square feet of solitude in which to entertain their muse and escape from the distractions of the world. To millions of people in the United States, Europe, and the Third World it is a privilege about which they dare not even dream.

That living alone should so often prove the occasions for loneliness and not the glorious opportunity for freedom and self-expression stems from the faulty logic we apply to the solitary situation: "I live alone, therefore I am lonely."

But try it this way: "I live alone, which means that I possess endless opportunities to enrich both my own life and the lives of others."

You Can:

Transform your room or apartment into the warm and vital center toward which gravitate friends, neighbors, colleagues in search of conversation, reassurance, sympathy, stimulation, amusement.

Run a "salon" and once a week or once a month invite people in who are strangers to each other to drink a cup of tea or a glass of wine, listen to records, read plays and discuss them, learn a language together. You become the catalyst in a host of new relationships, the friend in whom others confide.

Open your home to meetings of charity and political groups with which you are affiliated.

Open your home to a friend or colleague whose life will be brightened by a relaxing evening of talk.

Whatever the occasion, make your home the meeting place where others gather. (If you did not live alone, you would have to always consider whether it suited those with whom you live.)

You Can:

Live in many environments by changing you surroundings with the seasons—or when the mood strikes you. A can of paint, some inexpensive fabric, and a few prints picked up in a second hand shop can work wonders within your four walls.

Decorate your home to please a very important person: you. A small space facing on a back street can pulsate with warmth and beauty, and a manor house can send chills up your spine. It all depends on the attitude brought to the decorations.

Ask for advice. Millions of people do, otherwise decorators would go out of business. Invite a colleague or neighbor in and ask, "What would you do to this space?" The request will flatter your friend, and after you have asked a few, you will have acquired some good ideas.

Investigate other apartments or homes. Two things may happen: You may discover a perfectly delightful place and move within the month. Or you may return home blessing your good fortune and immediately begin refurbishing your present place, determined to realize all of its potential.

Tips on Living Alone

Freedom is exhilarating.

Its's fun to set your own schedule. But if you set no schedule, follow no regimen in your eating and exercise, your health will deteriorate along with your appearance.

Treat your home, whether it be one room, an apartment, or a large house, as the dynamic center of your life. Discover ways to add to its charm, develop its potential.

Change your surroundings occasionally. A new paint job, rearranging furniture, colorful posters and prints can bring an almost overnight chance.

Regularly open your home to others. The prospect of regular visitors enforces a healthy discipline in maintaining your surroundings. Even more important, your walls thereafter reverberate with the words, the problems, the happy presence of others.

Enjoy the freedom afforded by living alone. Don't abuse it cheaply by "letting go" of your grow-young regimens just because no one is watching.

Regenerating Sleep

Why is sleep important to your grow-young program? Because science tells us that body cells reproduce far more rapidly during deep sleep than when we are awake. So sleep is literally regenerating, "making you over," as it were, with its vital replenishment of cells. Without the right kind of sleep, your grow-young program cannot succeed.

Sleep that rests and refreshes, that nourishes the mind and the body, and prepares you to greet each day joyously and with renewed confidence in your powers is nature's great rejuvenator. In sleep, the wires of your life system that get crossed and mangled during the day—whether it be in the kitchen, on the job, or negotiating traffic on the throughway—straighten themselves out and plug in once more to your inner sources of strength, love, delight, and hope. As you awaken after a good night's sleep, life literally begins anew, regardless of chronological age.

The Sleep You Need

Have you ever laid awake worrying that you were not getting enough sleep?

Or slept ten to twelve hours and awakened more fatigued than when you retired?

Do you remember the time when you "worked like a dog" on cleaning the house or painting the bedroom and got up the next morning after only five or six hours sleep feeling as wide-awake and refreshed as a teen-ager at the start of vacation?

These apparent contradictions are not listed to confuse you about sleep but to help in getting rid of the "sleep superstitions" that may be blocking your own enjoyment of this wonderful gift of nature.

Fatigue alone, for example, is no sure indicator that you need more sleep than you are getting now. If it springs from dissatisfaction with your job or a family disagreement about how the budget should be handled, ten hours a night spent sleeping won't help you to shake off the feeling of tiredness. Sleep as a place to hide from your problems may offer temporary forgetfulness, but it contributes little to your relaxation and refreshment.

When you awake from a long, deep sleep feeling sapped of your energy and "tired before you start," look to the anxieties and frustrations, the boredom and the internal conflicts that may be troubling you rather than to overwork for the cause. Work you enjoy produces the blissful kind of relaxed tiredness that soon sends you off into refleshing sleep. But just the anticipation of an unwelcome task can cause you to wake in an apprehensive state where even the act of preparing breakfast or dressing for work may demand all your reserves of energy.

Some people worry themselves into continued wakefulness because they do not sleep a full eight hours every night. That they have been getting along marvelously on six hours at night and a nap in the daytime does not impress them. Of course the worry builds up, and the quality of their sleep gradually diminishes. Prisoners of the "sleep superstition," they turn from the gift that nature has given them to search for some impossible goal of "the right number of hours of sleep."

What few realize is that sleep is not a regimen with fixed rules suitable to all. It is an intensely personal kind of refreshment to which each individual must find his own individual key. Thomas A. Edison, for example, would work for long hours into the night without reducing his inventiveness or impairing his health. He had not conquered the need for sleep, however, but merely discovered the sleep pattern that worked for him. At his desk in the laboratory, on the couch in his office, he would drop off for an hour whenever he felt the need and awake refreshed and full of ideas.

The French writer Marcel Proust, when composing his immense novel, *Remembrance of Things Past,* would begin his "day" long after dark, dropping in at the late dinner parties of the social world he was so minutely chronicling and then working at his desk until far into the morning. One of the "great insomniacs," Proust transmuted his sleepless hours into the pure gold of creativity, producing one of the masterpieces of twentieth-century literature.

In the cities of Europe and America there are as many keys to relaxed sleep as there are hours. Doctors, policemen, firemen, trainmen, entertainers—these are just a few of the people who thrive on unconventional sleep patterns and have found ways to adjust the need for rest to the requirements of their jobs. Perhaps the most universal example of all, so common that it is seldom mentioned, is the mother who instantly awakes to the cry of her child whatever hour of the night yet still gets sufficient nourishing sleep.

Your Sleep Schedule

If there are no hard and fast rules, how can you tell if you are getting enough sleep? Doctors who have studied sleep deficiency list a number of indicators among them:

> A continuous feeling of tiredness, sometimes translated as "feeling a little older."
>
> A lack of self-confidence—you're not quite sure you can cope with dinner on Sunday when your in-laws are expected or you start dreading the prospect of a new assignment at the office.
>
> Your bridge or your golf game is not up to par, and you become irritable at the new clumsiness you display.
>
> You bump into the steps on the way upstairs and

misjudge the bottom step on the way down.

The cushions that protected you against the abrasions of everyday living seems to have worn thin. The screaming child down the street drives you up the wall or the homeward-bound traffic seems like a personal assault on your nerves.

You can multiply these instances by the thousandfold in your own life. What they spell out is "not enough sleep." It is better to heed these warning signals when they first appear because they can accumulate into serious hazards. Premature aging is one, with the evidence reflected not just by your mirror but by the glances thrown your way by family, friends, and co-workers. Your tense expression, the tightening of your muscles, the increasing susceptibility to resent unintended slights and to find offense where none is due, the shortness of temper that strikes out at your family, are just a few of the ways in which insufficient sleep takes its toll.

Your Better Sleep Program

Visit your doctor. The clean bill of health he gives you will at least assure you that your sleep problem is not organic; it seldom is.

Avoid being trapped by the "sleep superstition." Experiment with different sleep patterns. If you find difficulty getting seven or eight hours sleep in one stretch, try napping for an hour before lunch and again later in the afternoon. If you work all day, schedule your nap when you reach home in the evening. It may mean a late dinner–and a relaxed, enjoyable "continental" evening.

Stop worrying about sleep. Remember, the world is full of unconventional sleepers, and among them are many of the world's most creative people. If you have difficulty dropping off, just think of the prestigious company you are in—writers and artists and composers and businessmen and women who find in their "night thoughts" a major source of inspiration.

Place a notebook and tiny light by your bed. When you have a thought, write it down. You may find yourself waking from a half sleep several times in the early part of the night, but having emptied your mind of these thoughts, you will find yourself drowsing and falling into sleep with a happy sense of accomplishment. It beats trying to chase the thoughts from your mind or attempting to remember them the next day. Your "Night Book," incidentally, may turn up several creative suggestions that you can use in your work or conversation. Tapping a level of consciousness unavailable during the daytime hours, you will discover hidden areas of your personality.

This is *not* to say you should take problems to bed with you. There is a difference between accommodating and transferring to your "Night Book" thoughts that come to you unsolicited and gearing your mind and emotions for a tussle with major problems. In the first instance you place potentially disturbing thoughts outside of yourself, mentally acknowledging that they have been disposed of for the night. In the second case you deliberately ward off sleep and prepare for combat.

Surprise yourself one evening when you are feeling relaxed but not sleepy. Just go to bed an hour earlier. You may not immediately drop off, but neither will you worry about it. After all, it's early! So you have plenty of time to practice some sleep-inducing exercises—just for the fun of it.

Practice going to sleep in bits and pieces. Set the stage with a few minutes of deep, regular breathing. Then relax the muscles in one leg, the other leg; one arm and then the other. Follow through with your neck, your back, your thighs. Make it a pleasant experience, this bit by bit signing off from the day. Drifting on a gentle wave of gradual relaxation, submit to the developing "mood" of your body as it looses its hold on the daytime world. Await with quiet joy the refreshment and renewal that sleep will bring.

Discover sleep-inducing rituals that work just for you.

Some Things to Try

A lukewarm bath in which you relax for twenty minutes or half an hour.

Forget about television and the news and play some good records. "The magic of music is in its effect on volition," wrote one of our great modern poets. "There's a sudden clearing of the mind of rubbish and the re-establishment of a sense of proportion." And that's what you want to do before sleep—clear out the rubbish, get things in balance, and let go.

Keep a book by your bedside—not a thriller packed with violence but, if it's a novel, preferably the old-fashioned kind that goes on and on—a paperback edition of Jane Austen or Thackeray or Proust. Better still, reread some old favorite. You will be secure in the knowledge of what happens next and won't hesitate to close the book as you begin to drowse.

Food can aid in inducing sleep—if taken in moderation. A glass of warm milk is an all-time favorite—and while doctors may not recommend it, some find a small glass of port or sherry beneficial.

What about sleeping pills and barbiturates? Only if prescribed by the doctor. It is too easy to make a ritual of taking these products, which do nothing to build up life-enhancing sleep habits. If there is an underlying problem for sleeplessness, the pills merely camouflage it for a short while—and leave you with an even bigger problem to face later on.

Remember, you alone can discover your personal key to healthy sleep. Where or when you sleep is unimportant. If the sofa suits you better than the bed, if you feel more secure with the light on than in the darkness, if you sleep better in short spurts and can take cat-naps—well, why not?

To plunge joyously into sleep, to awake refreshed and alert to the challenge of a new day, is to experience, day in and day out, a true regeneration of yourself.

Sleep And Dreams

But sleep is more than nature's way of energizing your system for the tasks of the day. It is the gateway into a timeless world where you share with mankind the common heritage of myths and symbols. Here you plunge deep into pools of memory and retrieve the plunder of experience hidden from your waking eye—inestimable riches without which your existence would be threadbare indeed.

In your dreams, you explain, reconcile, or move onto another level the many contradictions that seem irreconcilable during the day. You set out on intense emotional adventures and summon up the kind of mental concentration on problems of which you would scarcely believe yourself capable. Pushing aside the walls of convention and inhibition that hem you in during the day, you release your creative self from captivity and extend the realms of what is possible to you.

Understandably, you may not always relish your dreams. Often they challenge the image that you have built for yourself—and confront you with a deeper reality you may not be prepared to acknowledge. But if you insist on banishing your dreams, you may pay a high price, for science is now revealing that nature intended these dream adventures as an integral part of what may be termed "creative sleep" or REM (rapid eye movement) sleep.

As you dream, these rapid eye movements are discernible beneath your closed lids, indicating an extreme degree of emotional and mental activity. Simultaneously, other physiological changes may be taking place, such as unusually rapid breathing, irregular heartbeats, and changes in your blood pressure. At the same time, some of your muscles may turn completely limp, accounting for the sense of helplessness that some dreamers experience. Scientists have called this combination of activities an "internal storm," and it certainly seems far removed from the picture of quiet, blissful sleep that you would look forward to at the end of the day. Yet, startling as it may seem, these upheavals form an important requisite of your night's rest—and it is when you are deprived of them that trouble sets in. Thus researchers have discovered that when sleepers are awakened at the start of their REM sleep, they start the next morning off in a state of fatigue and irritability, their normal ability to function significantly impaired. On nights succeeding the experiments, when permitted to sleep uninterrupted, they spend a longer than usual time in dreaming as signaled by rapid eye movement, as if to replenish their psychic economy with the food of dreams that had been denied to them.

Occurring at approximately one-and-a-half-hour intervals, REM sleep is nature's way of releasing the tensions you have built up during the day, of handling the emotional problems that may have remained repressed since childhood. It is a life-enhancing activity, your personal theater where you rewrite the drama of your past and present according to a script dictated by your deeper consciousness.

Deny or repress your dreams, and you cut yourself off from one of the profound sources of your humanity. For dreams bring to your waking hours an awareness of the poetry and mystery that surround your existence and that are all too often obscured by routine cares and worries. They are both a passport to the universal journey through life and the gateway to your own secret world.

Getting A Grow-Young Perspective On Sex and Romance

Nowhere in our personal lives does so much confusion reign as in the area of sexual relations.

Today we inhabit simultaneously a period of immense candor and enlightenment—and the dark ages.

Household magazines bring to their discussions of impotence, frigidity, and the liberated orgasm the same surface aplomb and sophistication that grace their glossy pages on decorating and design.

Yet twenty-five percent of the medical schools in the United States include no discussion of natural sex functions in their curriculum, and half the marriages in the country are troubled by some form of sexual problem, according to Masters and Johnson, the noted sex researchers.

Balanced precariously between knowing everything and understanding little indeed about this explosive force, we may be forgiven if we sometimes panic before its demands or seek to banish its troublesome presence from our lives.

Neither panic nor denial, however, will unlock the lasting sources of grow-young energy and vitality with which sex can infuse our lives, whether we be thrity-five or sixty-five. For that we need a new perspective, one that we must fashion out of our uniqueness and singularity as total human beings.

To isolate sex as a pleasure mechanism or as a test of our femininity or virility is to at once diminish its creative power and unleash its capacity for destruction. Only when we accord it a place in our lives as "part of the whole," along with work, involvement, play, peace of mind, consideration for others, and self-esteem, do we meaningfully connect with its mystery and delight and force for renewal.

Sexual Myths That Age Us—And How to Destroy Them:

It's Now or Never

Perhaps no message delivered by the sex researchers has been more important than the one that revealed that libido and sexual capability continue uninterrupted into the later years.

Once we comprehend that, given reasonably good health, there is no reason why we should not enjoy sexual relations well into our fifties and sixties (and beyond!), we rid ourselves of the destructive deadlines that haunt our thirties and forties.

Menopause does not spell the end of sexuality and the beginning of old age. Of course we can use it as an excuse for turning off on sex or for ceasing to care about our appearance, but another excuse would serve as well. What menopause does signal is the end of child-bearing, and for many women an end to the fear of pregnancy heralds a new era of freer and more enjoyable sex.

Similarly, the so-called male climacteric or "midlife crisis" does not bring impotence in its wake. Here, too, a hormonal change occurs, but the reasons for any diminishing of sexual desire at this time are far more psychological than biological. Worry, not incapacity, becomes the inhibiting factor–worry that perhaps potency is vanishing, that the body may have lost some of its desirability, that a temporary incapacity, perhaps triggered by a nagging problem at the office, may be the first sign of the dreaded loss of virility.

The myth that after thirty-five or forty-five the sexual road leads downhill all the way can panic us into an unhappy affair or turn a once-happy marriage into a veritable hell. Sometimes, rather than live with the uncertainty, we may simply turn our backs on the entire sexual situation, fleeing into obesity or alcoholism or overwork. We may even deliberately set about aging ourselves, withdrawing from life-enhancing involvement and abandoning all our health maintenance and grow-young programs.

And it is all so unnecessary. There is no cut-off year in our lives for sexual relations, no birthday after which desire and capability automatically vanish forever. So relax, take it easy. There is next week and next month and next year and the year after that. What you don't do today you can do tomorrow.

Conformity

Despite the much vaunted permissiveness of our times, we often conceive of sex in as tightly a regimented fashion as our Victorian forebears. Each age, it seems, enforces its own conformity, and ours is one of standards and averages. Thus we carry into the bedroom our mania for statistics, proof of performance, documentation.

Prisoners of the myth that there is an ideal statistical average of sexual activity, we grade ourselves accordingly. If we fall below the average, we begin to worry, plunging into frenetic activity, not because of an upsurge of desire but in order to prove that we can meet our quota.

Whatever positive energy we may have drawn from the sexual situation is dissipated in this negative pursuit of conformity. Even if we succeed in "upping" our performance under these adverse conditions, we achieve no lasting release from sexual anxiety. There is always next time to worry about.

So many times a week or month. Good, fair, poor . . . To rid ourselves of this obsession with standards and averages, we must reclaim our sexuality from the realm of performance and relocate it in the domain of personal feelings, where desire alone dictates activity.

The intervals and conditions under which we enjoy sexual relations may be as varied as our individual background, situation, physical condition, preferences, needs, and state of mind allow. Just as there is no such creature as "the average person," so there is no such phenomenon as average sexuality. Whatever is right for you, is right.

Make up your mind to drop out of the sexual sweepstakes today. Don't waste this tremendous force for life in what has to be a loser's game. Forget about the ratings and get back to the true sexuality that is uniquely your own.

The Proving Grounds

One of the most destructive myths of the day is that you prove your femininity or masculinity in bed. Competition replaces love, and the sexual relationship becomes tangled in a vicious web of economics, rivalries, and power drives. Everything is wagered on the ability to perform or respond. Each partner seeks his or her separate victory at the expense of mutuality of feeling and regard.

Our sexuality cannot hold up under the intolerable strain caused by this "all or nothing" confrontation, this repeated "putting it on the line." And the toll on the individual begins to show.

No lifetime of sexual acts could sum up the richness and

complexity of our total sexuality as men and women, which shines forth everyday in thousands of ways. To really "prove" our femininity or masculinity we would have to unravel the web of life itself and trace each strand back to the beginning of time.

Whatever hypothetical "victory" we may believe we gain in bed is tiny and insignificant indeed compared to the major ones we win day in and day out in the battle for survival. So let us abandon the destructive myth of the sexual proving grounds and move on to a tolerant and amused acceptance of ourselves, for with all our faults and limitations and idiosyncrasies we are still quite wonderful.

Sex Is Everywhere

True—and false.

The erotic impulse infuses all of life, fom birth to death. It is in the *Song of Songs,* the poetry of Shakespeare, in Bach's Brandenburg Concerti. It infuses religion, architecture, and the arrangements we make for living together as a society. But it is present not only as subject and theme but as a life force, the drive behind the creativity of the masters and the generator that powers our own day-to-day achievements.

Sex as transcendent power, energy, force, informed the lives of men centuries before the "sex culture" exploded on the scene. Paradoxically, our present conception of sex as a sexual relationship in the obvious sense really constitues a narrowing and diminishing of this life force. There is more to sex than sex-in-bed.

We tap our sexual resources in our work, our sports, our play, in building a business, in community work, in extending kindness to others, and in our moments of quiet and contemplation.

The power of sex brings a warmth separate from desire to our relationships with friends and colleagues of all ages. It glows beneath the surface of platonic romances and kindles a gathering of strangers momentarily brought together by accident or circumstances. Sexuality, then, is a measure of our common humanity.

Let us refuse to accept the media limitation on sex as exclusively the expression of desire between individuals. Certainly and wonderfully it is that. But let us acknowledge it also as the source of infinite power and creativity and sympathy throughout every moment of our lives.

More Is Better

We live in an economy of abundance. Every day we are solicited to want more, buy more, use more. It is not surprising that the myth of "more is better" should color our sex lives and that we should seek to increase the number of our sexual partners.

The pursuit of quantity, however, has nothing to do with desire or sexuality. It is acquisitiveness. And endless pursuit of acquisitions is wearying and aging.

To change sex partners because of love or desire or incompatibility is one thing. To keep changing because we seek some unattainable answer to all of our problems is something else.

Sexuality expands as a force for growing young from a continuing relationship, one in which we take the time to explore the other as a total human being, body, mind, emotions, hopes, fears. Out of this profound human contact springs the sense of refreshment and happiness that brings a lilt to our voice, a buoyancy to the way we walk, a youthful glow to our cheeks.

Romance Is Dead

Candlelight, music, wine, soft clothes, and perfume–relics of a bygone era. Or are they? Gradually we are learning to touch one another again, to hold hands as we walk down the street, to lean on a shoulder as we listen to music, to show affection.

Romance, that maligned term, is returning, carried into our lives on a current wave of nostalgia but touching responses that endure beyond the moment.

At any and every age, we should find a place for romance in our lives—for romantic occasions at home, for flirtations, for the glance and the word that tells another that we recognize and appreciate their singularity as man or woman.

Yes, we must destroy the negative myths that distort sexuality and deprive it of its full dimension in our lives. But we must restore the positive myths that bring color and beauty into our lives. Without romance, we "have sex" but we do not make love.

Helping One Another

Where do you go for help with a sex problem?

Teen-agers and young marrieds can at least talk it out among themselves. After thrity it's not that easy.

The classic answer is to your doctor, minister, or psychiatrist.

But it's the rare doctor who has the time to do anything more than work on any physical roadblocks to sexual fulfillment.

And while the minister may offer solace, he seldom has the ability to handle the sexual hang-ups that plague so many individuals today.

The importance of the psychiatrist in helping with real emotional problems should not be underestimated. But sexual fulfillment is an interrelated phonomenon and not a thing in itself.

So often the resolution of the problem lies within the situation—and that means between you and your sex partner. For it is a case of "my problem is your problem" and vice versa. No two people have more of a vested interest in coming up with a solution.

In many relationships sex is a topic that is just not discussed, no matter how serious the problem. When such a communications barrier exists attacking it head-on seldom works.

But it is possible to open up the channels of communication about sex by increasing your communication in all other areas. This is "setting the stage," and it produces an atmosphere in which one topic can develop into another and another—and indirectly lead to an examination of the sexual problem.

The biggest asset in any such discussion is acceptance and tolerance. Recall the statistics quoted at the beginning of this chapter: Approximately half the marriages in this country are troubled by sexual problems. You and your sex partner are two of millions. This realization alone should remove some of the pressure.

Undoubtedly a big percentage of those problems are worse than yours. Aceepting the fact of "all of us are in the same boat," try at first for small improvements. Don't try to fix blame because in these situations few of us are without fault. We each have our hang-ups that the other must tolerate.

Strive for mutuality of regard: I will tolerate you if you will tolerate me. Accept the other's idiosyncrasies and gently suggest that the other accept yours.

Talk—and touch, which conveys acceptance, reassurance, love.

Enhance the opportuninities for sexual fulfillment with attention to health, cleanliness, grooming, rest, exercise, and diet and all the other grow-young practices suggested in this book.

Admire and appreciate your body. Only then can another desire you. And bring romance into your life. Candlelight, music, perfume are as important at forty and fifty and sixty as at twenty-five.

Fatigue, distraction, unrealistic expectations, can bar the road to pleasure. So choose your time for love when they have been banished.

Because sex is so closely associated with the fountain of youth, we sometimes look for magic potions and spells that would assure us of enduring potency and desire. But to waste our time in fantasies is to miss the true magic of sexuality, which is yours to enjoy here and now.

We grow young through living our days to the fullest and not wasting one of them.

A Time for Quiet

There is a time for action—and a time for stillness, for putting aside the unrelenting busy-ness of everyday living and finding our way back to the center of our being where dwell peace of mind, a joy independent of circumstances, and a youthful spirit unimpaired by chronological age.

Where and how we make these moments of quiet is unimportant. We can enjoy them walking alone in the rain through a deserted city street, watching a sunset from a rooftop, or beside a lake, fishing rod in hand. Alone in our room, we may stretch out motionless on the floor or rise early in the morning, and while everyone is alseep, sit quietly experiencing the dawn, mind completely free of the ambitions and pretensions of the acquisitive world.

The moments pass, but the sense of profound well-being they bring to us remains. Without making room for these centers of stillness in our lives, our senses, our perception of good and evil, our ability to experience the sheer joy of living, diminishes.

Distractions, not adversity, engraves the haggard, nervous look on so many of the faces we pass in the streets today. With our attention solicited a million and one different ways, we wear ourselves out responding helter-skelter to random stimuli that hold neither meaning nor pleasure for us.

Activities, amusements, desires, participation in the rich and turbulent life of the world today, these form legitimate and necessary parts of our lives. But once a day we must muster the courage to cry, "Enough! This time belongs to me."

Conceive of these moments of stillness as the occasion for rebirth, in which the self shucks off the anxieties, frustrations, and bothersome cares accumulated during the day and emerges purified, refreshed, once more in touch with the harmony of the self and the universe.

During these precious intervals of quiet and absorption, hang-ups dissolve and tensions vanish, along with their visible evidence: the clamped jaw, drawn mouth, furrowed brow, and upset stomach. The body "lets go" of its compulsive hold on worldly structures; commands, defenses, schedules recede into the distance. The senses open out, and we experience with heightened awareness the slightest movement of air on our skin, the hidden nuances in a phrase of music. We are both at peace with the world and wondrously alive.

Rituals for Peace

Rituals for achieving quietude are best performed alone. At first you will need some preparatory time to ease yourself into this state of pure consciousness. Start by physically slowing down and literally washing away the evidence of the day's barrage on your nerves and senses. When you get home, instead of turning on television or reading the mail, prepare a leisurely bath, not just an in-and-out shower. Submerge yourself in a tub as though you were floating off the coast of some island. Play a Mozart quartet on the record player and remain in the tub until it is finished. Then dry leisurely and anoint your body with cologne or oils and, with the lights turned low, or with the sunlight shining in on you, stretch out full length, perhaps on the floor instead of your bed.

One at a time, slowly tense your muscles and just as slowly relax them. First one hand, then the other. Curl up the toes of one foot as tightly as possible and then slowly let go. Now do the same thing with the other. Stretch one arm at a time, one leg, tighten your buttocks and slowly let go. Tense every muscle until you have gone through the entire bodily repertoire of holding in and letting go: tension, release; tension, release; tension, release until every muscle feels soothed.

Now breathe deeply, hold your breath and then exhale slowly, all the way until you have cleared your lungs of all the air you took in. Repeat this deep and slow breathing six times.

While you are making these preparations, focus you mind on your bodily sensations. Bit by bit, the thought patterns of the day will begin to dissolve into fragments. As your body unlearns the right-left, first-this-step, now-that-step programming by which it functions in the workaday world, so your mind relinquishes its hold on the ambitions, plans, woes, the daily store of anxieties and grievances and pressures. Mentally and physically, you clear the way for the moments of stillness and undistracted quiet.

Lie perfectly still for fifteen minutes. Don't attempt to keep track of time. If you like, set an automatic timer to go off after that interval, or just lie there for as long as you feel the need.

It is not communing with a spiritual force that you are seeking. although there may be a comparison. Rather it is quietude and peace within oneself. At one with ourselves, our bodies, nerves, emotions, and minds are renewed, dissolved, reunited and at peace with the other.

Accustomed as we are to having our mind jump all over the place, most of us have to discipline our thoughts at the outset with the aid of a "control" word or thought. Focus your mind on a word, a musical sound or scene that suggests solitude and peace. Perhaps the slow, rhythmic repetition of a phrase will empty your mind of distractions, or you may recall and hold in mind a waterfall glimpsed while walking through the woods, a tiny walled garden that seemed like an enclave of blissful solitude amidst the bustle of the city. A mockingbird concert you heard years ago, or an organ prelude. Or a flower you bought on the way home.

Many people find softly played music helpful in blocking out other sounds and in clearing the mind of the cares and details that stubbornly refuse to go away.

The flicker of a candle or firelight, a ritual cup of tea, the touch of a polished stone or wood that is old and worn and warm.

Try several mood-setting approaches and use the one that works for you. Remember, however, that your objective is consciousness divorced of everyday concerns and at a spiritual level to which we do not ordinarily attain. Sleep is not the goal.

Relaxed, absorbed in your consciousness of peace and quietude, you are still, pulled neither this way nor that, at the center of your being. You desire only this, being is enough.

Do not expect to achieve a complete absence of distracting thoughts the first or second time. Some of us never achieve total peace, but that does not diminish our rewards. The more expert we become through practice in letting go of the world, the more we will treasure these moments of stillness from which we return refreshed and renewed in body and spirit.

After a few sessions, you will find the elaborate preparations for turning off the world becoming unnecessary. A part of yourself, attuned to stillness and quiet being, anticipates these moments and begins to slow down your mental and physical clock as the expected time approaches. In the middle of a busy day, with the sounds of children or cars or television sets at their loudest, you can still turn inward and connect with a world in which there is quiet and peace, free of pressures to do, react, respond to the demands of others.

The Need to Be Alone

We "make up" our faces and our minds to impress others. Like actors, we are always on stage, responding to cues written into the drama of our lives by circumstances. With a wide repertory of "body language" we convey desire, rejection, anticipation, pleasure, pain, and all the messages of which we are humanly capable.

Alone we continue to wear our mask, for we, too, are spectators at our own drama as well as actors. Only in sleep is it removed and then only partially, for often we continue to play our roles in dreams with even greater resolve and abandon.

The time of stillness is one way of getting off stage for a few moments and maintaining contact with our unique selves. Positive use of a few carefully cultivated moments of solitude in each day is another.

Life offers no greater reward than true sharing of our joys and pains with another. But unless we bring to this sharing the oneness with self garnered during our solitude, the contribution we make may be meager indeed compared to our potential for sharing.

When we go off by ourselves for a walk down a country road or through the city streets, we are not rejecting the other, but enriching the self that the other shares. Each day, we need these few moments of solitude to "get ourselves together," to take off the mask and ungarble our lines.

There are many small ways in which we can ease ourselves out of our workaday roles.

Ways to Spend Your "Quiet Time"

Walk part of the way home alone. Before dinner, stroll through the street for twenty minutes. Or just go to your room and stretch out on the floor.

Make the transition from office or housework a significant one. Bathe leisurely, change into comfortable, colorful clothes and, if you live with another, relax with some special project of your own, or with a book in a room alone.

Stand in front of a mirror and slowly stretch, stretch, stretch your head and arms as high as you can. Then lightly run your fingers over your forehead, face, neck, slowly and deliberately, several times, removing the mask of every day.

Make time in the early morning to work on a private project or plan that is relaxing and diverting and is not tied up with your work or usual concerns.

Spend a few minutes on a different kind of speech. Read aloud from an anthology of poetry, or dip into some volume of prose from an earlier century.

Surround yourself for an evening with your favorite collection of objects: fabrics, books, antique buttons, theater programs, colored glass.

Keep a diary. Each day, in a room alone, record your impressions, thoughts, desires, the joy you experience and the anguish. Be yourself, not polite or "literary," and if you can't stand your boss or want to move to a different community to get away from an obtrusive neighbor, say so. This is your private world.

Create. Painting, needlework, writing, woodworking, crafts of all kinds, enable us to be alone, to collect our thoughts or just "let go" while we disconnect the world and reconnect with ourselves through creative actions. Those of us who have set aside a tiny section of our living quarters where we can "create" undistracted and free from the demands of role-playing are fortunate indeed.

The rewards of learning to be at peace with ourselves and making the time for it are enormous: Our health, looks, confidence and patience with others perceptibly improve. We age through distraction, and the endless random stimuli of daily living pulls us one way and another, without direction or purpose.

In quietude, in the creative use of solitude, we find our selves and our way, beneath the ambitions and frustrations, to a level of consciousness and being where we experience again the true harmony of existence.

Putting Retirement in Its Place

Retirement is one of those ambivalent words that are fraught with different meanings for different individuals. Some of us look forward to it with the same youthful anticipation of freedom and adventure with which we approached graduation day. Released from the demands of the job, we will finally possess the time and the space to enjoy our lives.

To others, the word "retirement" sounds the death knell of all that is worthwhile in life. We see stretching before us interminable years of idleness during which no one will call upon our talent, our skills, or indeed any of our human resources. The prospect is bleak indeed as we contemplate the fate of 10 percent of the population turned into economically and socially stateless persons by this arbitrary termination of our working lives.

What gives retirement its special urgency, regardless of whether we look forward to it with joy or dread, is the increasingly lower age at which it is encountered. Absurd as it may seem, hale and hearty men and women are forced into idleness at a time when they are really approaching the peak of their powers. Just as their experience, confidence, and accumulated wisdom start to pay off, management lowers the boom.

Officially, a corporation may set a retirement age at sixty or sixty-five. In actuality, many begin enforcing retirement in the forties and fifties through selective hiring practices. In the United States, Britain and on the continent, many executives who lose their jobs in the mid-forties find that for all practical purposes they have been "retired" from the job market—and without a pension—because they can no longer find positions at the same level of salary or responsibility.

Nor is management the only culprit. Increasingly the labor unions, under pressure to admit more young members and find jobs for them, agitate for lower retirement ages, the theory being that the more older workers they can remove at the top of the scale, the more younger workers they can find jobs for at the bottom.

Thus it can be seen that the so-called "youth culture," with its adulation of everyone under thirty and its despair of everyone over, is supported by a firm economic base. And as the impact of automation grows, so will the push for earlier and earlier retirement.

Facing the Facts

Whether you are thirty-five, forty-five, or fifty-five, therefore, retirement has to figure into your grow-young program. How you conceive of it, how you plan for it, in what spirit you encounter it, these are the important questions to be decided. For the unprepared individual, retirement can prove a tragic aging experience, sapping energy, self-confidence, and the will to live. Almost overnight, deterioration sets in—and it can occur at forty-five as well as at sixty-five.

But retirement can also provide the occasion for tremendous self-renewal. One friend had been anticipating retirement for several years, and the day after leaving his office for the last time could be found happily engaged in the little at-home business he had looked forward to for so many years. That he relished his new freedom and new work was obvious in the way he bounced down the street, smiled at friends, and in the flair with which, each day, he attached a flower to his lapel, something he could not do at his old job. "I didn't retire," he rightly explains. "I finally shook free of that dreary job and got into something I really enjoy. And believe me, I'm working harder than ever." He is, too, and thriving on it.

Another couple did not wait until they were forced out of their jobs, but took advantage of an early retirement plan to move to Vermont and open a small business that they run with no other help. Now they find themselves rising early in the morning, full of energy and eager to get to work. They have recaptured a sense of excitement and challenge that they thought had disappeared forever. "We feel younger than we have in fifteen years," they report.

What this couple and thousands of others disprove with their resurgent second careers and enduring vitality is the immoral myth that men and women become useless after a certain age, that by the age of fifty or sixty or seventy, the individual's responses to the challenge of life diminish in force and sharpness, that he or she loses interest in issues, ideas, sex, and interaction with society. So the first thing to realize when encountering retirement is that it is a social and financial concept engineered to make jobs for younger workers. It is not a physical and psychological blight that descends on you overnight when you reach "retirement age," suddenly depriving you of your faculties, personality, sex drive, talents, and capabilities.

Otto Klemperer, the German-born conductor, retired from the New Philharmonic Orchestra of London at eighty-seven—but was careful to add that he would continue to conduct for recordings! Jacques Lipchitz, the master sculptor, continues to work, although he is past eighty, or, as he puts it, four times twenty. As Picasso approaches ninety, collectors and museums eagerly await his newest creations. In every village and city you will find men and women leading full and vigorous lives in their seventies and eighties, giving the lie to a society that, if it had its way, would have consigned them to the scrap heap twenty years ago.

Retirement may force you out of your job. Retirement cannot force you to relinquish your claim to the good things of life.

Whether or not you continue to grow young during retirement depends on the actions you take in your forties and fifties. Ralph Waldo Emerson, the New England sage, wrote that "We do not count a man's years until he has nothing else to count." And that about sums up successful retirement: having something else to count other than your years. Study those who have successfully negotiated society's arbitrary retirement age and you will find individuals who are active, concerned, committed, and involved. While they may have retired from a particular job, they certainly have not retired from life. They continue to lead constructive and rewarding lives that are rich in new experiences and interests.

Many of the restraints and inhibitions imposed by job situations have been lifted, and for the first time since youth, they discover that it is possible to indulge their tastes and fantasies freely. Restraints and responsibilities are fewer, opportunities and options are multiplied, and the psychological space for maneuvering grows more extensive.

Prisoners of the Myth

Why, then, do not more of us look forward to retirement with joyous expectancy rather than with resignation or dread?

In America and Britain in particular, we are prisoners of the work ethic. Our job defines our social status, value to society, self-esteem. When we meet a stranger, we ask, not "Who are you? What are your interests?" but "What do you do?" A woman may hook strikingly handsome rugs—but still define herself as a housewife. A man may have spent years building a collection of rare old bottles or antique prints and yet define himself as a welder or a sales manager.

Preparing for successful retirement means first of all getting away from the work definition of ourselves into one that is fuller, more rounded, and diverse and that does justice to the true richness of our lives. Obviously we cannot accomplish this transformation the day before retirement. This kind of re-evaluation of ourselves should begin in our forties and fifties (or sooner) as part of our stock-taking. Gradually, we push back the walls that narrow our perspective and restrict our actions and discover there is a whole world out there awaiting our enjoyment. Tentatively, we take the first few steps, sampling this treasure and then another, stopping to linger where we are attracted most. As we become interested, we find ourselves responding to stimuli in new ways. Enthusiasm bathes us in its warm glow. And we get busy, building interest(s) into our lives.

Our society so stresses professionalism on the job that we have forgotten the contributions to civilization of the amateur. The amateur gardener, woodcarver, mechanic, decorator, political activist, writer, both gives and receives lasting pleasure. He or she is never at a loss for something to do or say, and when the amateur retires from the workaday job, it is with the joyful anticipation of more time for carving, collecting, or whatever.

In our chapter on "Grow-Young Action Projects," we open up a few areas in which you might discover interests that will bring renewal into your life. In the best sense of the word, these are interests that can grow into full-time activities after technological retirement. In the amateur interests that they developed in their forties and fifties, people frequently find the sources of the small businesses they open in their sixties.

One of the major apprehensions that we experience when approaching retirement is that of "not being needed." After years of being in continuous demand on the job, suddenly the phone stops ringing, the tension snaps with startling swiftness, and we are left floating uneasily in a vacuum. If prolonged, this sensation can translate itself into fears about our capability to function as full human beings, and these fears in turn block the channels of self renewal. It is the ideal situation to encourage the onset of illness or premature age.

When we have interests to sustain us, however, and are not totally dependent on the job for psychological support, we can weather this transition nicely. Indeed, then it is upon retirement that we experience this surge of renewal, this realization that we have now attained a new level of experience in which we are enviably free—not to do nothing, but to do more of the things we find enjoyable and meaningful.

Never let the word "retirement" define your life. It signifies withdrawal, and anyone who withdraws from life at age sixty or sixty-five, barring serious illness (which can occur at any age), is undeserving of the rich, full existence that is part of our heritage.

Instead, define your new life by action: "I am a carpenter, I work at macrame, I garden. I am an activist in community affairs, a collector, a secretary, a woodsman, philosopher, nurse; I make clothes for the needy, teach the underprivileged to read, repair antique furniture, photograph the morning dew." These are your active interests, the doors that continuously open out onto new vistas, new friends, new challenges.

To repeat:

Retirement is a social condition, not a mental or physical one. You are just as capable of performing a task after retirement as before.

Become an amateur in the best sense of the word. Whatever your age, fill your life with interests outside your job. If your job is so satisfying and all-encompassing that you desire no other activity, then search for alternative means of performing it. A friend of mine had for twenty years worked for a company that built boats. When he retired, he moved to a lakeside communtiy and set up a small repair shop where he serves the needs of his neighbors.

Reread the chapter on "The Magic of Change." The more often you encounter change in your daily life, the easier it will be to negotiate the change brought by retirement.

The Positive Approach to Retirement

Retirement is a beginning. It is a time for action, for using your new-found free time to put more into life and to get more out of it. It is not a time for slowing down, for letting go, for giving up.

It is also a time for vigilance if you are to escape the silken traps set for the retired by society. Were it not tragic, the ideal image of the sixty-five-and-over man and woman given by television and in print would be farcical. There he or she is, sitting in a chair, wrapped up in memories and only occasionally bestowing a benign smile on the real world as it passes by. The individual who settles into that caricature of a human being soon becomes it: uninvolved, uninterested, uninteresting, without sex and without spirit, slowly atrophying into useless material for time's scrap heap.

Fear of retirement can start to age a person in the forties as they see the day approaching when the job props of their existances will be knocked from under them. In panic, they strike out blindly for escape: into alcohol, love affairs, rash financial ventures. Since none of these panic reactions bring a solution, they merely accentuate their distress and their inability to manage retirement when it arrives. This is the negative approach, and it is, unfortunately, the one that is reinforced by the attitudes of our society.

Renewal is a word that recurs again and again in this book. Look to it again for your key to positive retirement. We have talked about the importance of active projects in preparing for retirement. Now let us talk about activist attitudes for renewal.

Activist attitudes help us to break the sterotyped retirement image and to be ourselves. When we continue to be active and involved, we count for something more than our years. And since people tend to take us at our own estimation, the opportunities for action and involvement proliferate. Because we have some place to go, some mission to accomplish, we stride with our head up and shoulders back. Because we hearken to our bodies and not the anti-life platitudes of the image-makers, we continue to enjoy good food and good conversation, sex and the myriad sensations afforded by color, music, nature, movement.

It does take courage to "be yourself" after sixty-five. But consider for a moment: When before did you enjoy so much freedom! The demands of the job no longer impose a specific dress code, and if you want to sport a colorful pair of pants or ascot, to ride a bicycle to and from the shops, to go off by yourself on a cruise, who is to say no? If you have children, they are old enough to take care of themselves, and if you are alone, your friends can learn to put up with your individuality.

"When I retire, I plan to—" These are magic words, bespeaking a commitment to renewal and action and infusing energy into your system today and tomorrow. You may plan to get more involved politically, in the running of your town, in a volunteer community news service, in your specific interest.

You may plan to open a small business or join with others in a nonprofit educational program to transmit your skills to others. You may plan to take another job in a field that has always fascinated you.

For most of us, planning involves money, and there is no hiding the fact that, with few exceptions, retirement incomes prove inadequate to our needs. Right here we have another reason for adopting activist attitudes toward the after-retirement years—now. In our forties and fifties we can map out financial strategies that will build bridges between job and retirement and enable us to continue to lead constructive lives.

Happy indeed is the individual who plans retirement in such a way that amateur interests mesh with economic reality, so that the same amateur interest that provides life-renewing involvement also yields an income. Not everyone can achieve this happy blend, but we can all combine activist attitudes with sound planning in such a way as to enjoy the maximum amount of freedom possible in our particular situations.

When do you begin to plan? Today.

What Steps do You Take?

Realize that the way the economy is structured, chances are you will face retirement sometime between fifty-five and sixty-five. Realize, too, that the retirement years need not fall into the stereotyped pattern but can yield excitement, enjoyment, adventure, and income.

Put retirement in its place. Keep in mind that it does not signal a falling off of your mental and physical powers, which remain every bit as good after retirement as they did before, if you continue to use them, but that it is an arbitrary job cut-off by the system. Economically it may make sense. Psychologically and physiologically it is absurd.

Think of your life as a continuum. While your job supports this continuum up until retirement, you will have to support it afterward. Since it takes time to build these supports, start today.

Build on interests outside your job. After retirement these interests will flourish and expand.

Explore ways in which your interests can yield a supplementary income. The time to read up on the markets for your products and services, on merchandising techniques and costs and restrictions, is now, not a few months before you plan to open a shop or become a consultant in cost-saving. With this kind of planning you avoid the hazards of investing your money unwisely, of committing your funds at a time when you may have less flexibility than you enjoy with your present income.

Plan a renewal income for the retirement years. That

> could mean doing without a few things today, increasing your savings or investing small amounts in property or interest-yielding securities. This will not seem a deprivation when you keep in mind that additional income will provide the necessary fuel to maintain your interests in the future.
>
> Never slacken your campaign to introduce new beginnings into your life. New friends, new interests, new places.
>
> Some of us plan to move out of the city when we retire. But don't rule out the reverse. Increasingly, people not tied down by jobs and family are abandoning the suburbs and taking convenient apartments in town, which are near theaters, shops, and centers of activity. Whichever you plan, begin exploring the new territory now, even though retirement may be years away.

There are two reasons for this previewing activity. One is that you get to know the climatic and social conditions over a period of time. You discover whether or not the location will encourage your interests, whether you will feel at home, whether it has the kind of resources you require to lead a full life.

The second reason is that previewing helps maintain the continuum we were discussing before. You're less likely to fall for the myth that as soon as you retire you require coddling, a "soft" environment, absense of challenge and stress—in other words, what is known as "a retirement community."

Search for a community, and plan to live in the city or the suburbs that appeals to your abiding interests and drives, not in those distorted and artificial communities that are falsely supposed to characterize you when you reach the age of retirement.

Look for sources of renewal, not of stagnation.

Whatever you do, avoid retirement ghettos, however golden they may appear. Continue to cultivate new acquaintances of all ages, to share the interests of the young and to keep your mind open to new ideas. Do not permit others to impose their negative ideas of retirement on you and thus block off your sources of grow-young material. These are your years of freedom and action, too precious to be lifted arbitrarily out of the mainstream of life.

Remember: Action, change, and renewal are the conditions of growth and life. Yes, even in retirement—especially in what "they" call retirement!

Science and Growing Young

Had you been born in 1850, your life expectancy would have been between thirty-five and forty years.

Today it is about seventy, and a number of experts see the life span for many reaching to between seventy-five and one hundred years. Right now the United States has over five thousand individuals who have passed the one hundred-year mark. And as scientists explore further the potentialities of biochemistry, pharmacology, endocrinology, and of developing spare parts for the human body, we may come to expect increased longevity as part of our natural heritage.

While the sophisticated technology we now bring to research is comparatively recent, dating mostly from the period following World War II, interest in developing means of controlling the aging process and extending the life span gained considerable attention and support in the last quarter of the nineteenth century, sparked by the increasing knowledge about the action of hormones.

In France, Serge Voronoff attempted to achieve rejuvenation by transplanting animal glands into humans. Eugen Steinach, a noted researcher in the physiology of sex, turned his attention in the early 1920s to what he believed to be the rejuvenating effects of hormones produced by stimulation of the sex glands. Both efforts captured the attention of the medical world and the public at large for a time, but when no scientific proof of durable achievements could be produced, interest in these techniques collapsed.

Just as controversial among medical authorities but supported by staunch testimonials from some eminent and satisfied beneficiaries is the ongoing work in cellular therapy associated with Paul Niehaus, a Swiss surgeon, and the Montrose Clinic. The "rejuvenation" of Winston Churchill, Konrad Adenauer, and Somerset Maugham has been attributed to the work of Niehaus, which has as its basis the implantation by injection of cells taken from the organs of embryonic sheep. Basic to this form of cellular therapy is the assumption that the injected cells continue to live after injection and thus are able to carry out their rejuvenating work.

As with Voronoff and Steinach, the work of Niehaus lacks acceptance by the majority of the medical community, who point to the lack of clinical evidence or even verifiable reports of scientifically-controlled experiments. In addition to being very expensive, the rejuvenation treatments at the Montrose Clinic in Switzerland are available only to a few.

Medically approved and available to everyone for whom they are deemed advisable are the sex hormones, estrogen, testosterone, and progesterone. We all manufacture them in our bodies for a while. However, as the years pass, we cease to produce them, and the effects of this deficiency become apparent in ways that we associate with aging: poor posture, sagging skin, poor mental attitude. Thus many doctors prescribe them to female patients to alleviate menopausal problems and to help them retain their femininity. In that sense, they may be said to contribute to a "grow-young" effect. Whether or not the sex hormones can retard aging to a greater degree remains to be determined.

Science has already gone far in the development of vaccines to combat infections, and massive research continues on the number one killer, heart disease. Increasingly sophisticated mechanical devices such as heart valves and pacemakers are already in extensive use, and drugs to reduce blood pressure also contribute to the longevity of individuals once condemned to an inactive existence at best.

A new technique for combating disease called immunotherapy also holds promise. It mobilizes the patient's own resources against attack.

But perhaps for those of us concerned with growing young today the greatest promise of longevity comes from the new screening procedures designed to detect disease before it takes hold. Many of the indicators picked up by these tests yield to correction at an early stage so that the human system never experiences the aging effects of the disease.

Finally, we have within our own control a marvelous weapon for extending our years, and that is avoidance of the traps that age us. We know that if we watch our weight we have a better chance at a long and productive life than if we let go and put on extra pounds.

We know that if we continue to exercise and stay active we increase our chances of a healthy body that will endure for years.

We know that if we relinquish smoking we can increase our longevity odds significantly.

Indeed, throughout this book you have read of the need for maintenance, for action, and for purpose in each of the days of life.

But longevity itself should not be our goal. For some, the years drag interminably. No, we should pursue the goal of a life that is vigorous, involved, loving, and generous, giving to each day as much as we can and taking from it all the joys and challenges it offers.

We cannot just preserve our youth. If we attempt to do so, we will be caught on the sidelines, watching life rush by, which is a sure invitation to premature age.

But we can continue to grow and develop and rejoice in the possession of a youthful spirit that transforms the way we look and think and feel and live. This is truly "growing young."